Keto Meal Plan

Comprehensive 30 Day Ketogenic Diet Meal Plan With Handpicked Mouthwatering Ketosis-Inducing Recipes

Faith Smith

Introduction

If you have ever found yourself in a conversation where weight loss, optimum health and dieting were discussed, chances are you have heard about the Ketogenic diet. This is because it is the most talked about dietary plan in the world today. The reason why the ketogenic diet is so popular is that it is one of the best diets when it comes to health improvement and weight loss.

But as beneficial as ketogenic diet is, quite a number of people who adopt it (including myself) fail to benefit from it because of one simple reason; we simply eat the same old meals and don't plan our meals. So what happens when following the diet; we get bored eating the few keto meals that we know how to make and we give up on our commitment to the diet.

This happened to me quite a bit and I found myself not sticking to the diet. However, I was very committed and I knew where the problem was; therefore, I started experimenting with different meals and over time came up with some Keto-friendly meals that I love.

In this book, I share delicious and mouth-watering keto recipes that will not only make you enjoy following the keto diet but will also make the people around you want to adopt the diet too.

In this guide, you will have adequate recipes to last you up to 30 days or even more. This 30-day meal plan is designed to help you achieve your health and fitness goals as effortlessly as possible.

However, before you get to learn the 30-day program and recipes, you will first be introduced to ketogenic diet where you will learn:

- What it is

- How it works

- Reasons why you should try it

- How you can get started on it

- And lots of other important stuff that will get you started and hold you by the hand throughout the process

So without further ado, let us get started.

PS: Don't forget to leave a review of this book on Amazon if you are happy with it.

Table of Contents

Introduction---2

About The Author----------------------------------- 11

The Basics: Ketogenic Diet For Beginners --12

What Is A Ketogenic Diet? ------------------------- 12

How A Ketogenic Diet Works---------------------- 12

Signs Of Being In A State Of Ketosis ------------- 16

Is Keto Diet For Everyone? ------------------------ 17

Why The Ketogenic Diet? --------------------- 19

Getting Started ------------------------------------ 25

Step 1: Know The Right Amount Of
Macronutrients To Take----------------------------25

Step 2: Learn What To Eat And What Not To Eat
--- 28

Step 3: Go Out For Shopping And Kick Start The
Diet--31

Breakfast Recipes-------------------------------- 33

Keto Rolls---33

Keto Frittata ---------------------------------------36

Chorizo Omelette ----------------------------------- 38

Blueberry Smoothie ------------------------------- 41

Baked Mini-Frittatas ----------------------------- 42

Breakfast Biscuit Sandwiches --------------------- 44

Cauliflower Hash Browns-------------------------- 46

Keto Breakfast Cheesecake ----------------------- 48

Bacon Cheeseburger Waffles --------------------- 51

Blueberry Coconut Porridge---------------------- 54

Egg-Crust Pizza ---------------------------------- 56

Basic Oopsie Rolls ------------------------------- 58

Cream Cheese Pancake --------------------------- 60

Breakfast Roll Ups------------------------------- 61

Breakfast Salad --------------------------------- 63

Brie & Apple Crepes ----------------------------- 66

Avocado Egg Bowls------------------------------- 68

Keto Breakfast Quiche --------------------------- 70

Sausage Gravy and Biscuit Bake ----------------- 72

Pumpkin Spice Latte ----------------------------- 75

Crustless Quiche--------------------------------- 77

Coconut Cream With Berries --------------------- 79

Lunch Recipes ----------------------------------80

Eggplant and Beef Casserole-------------------- 80

Lasagne Stuffed Portobello ---------------------- 82

Taco Bowls with Cauliflower Rice---------------- 84

Pork Skewers with Chimichurri ----------------- 86

Keto Tortang Talong------------------------------ 88

Cheesy Zucchini Aglio E Olio --------------------91

Grilled Turkey Burger ---------------------------93

Chicken with Radishes and Spinach -------------95

Dill Pickle Soup --------------------------------97

Caramelized Onion Croquettes Stuffed with Goat Cheese--- 99

Coleslaw-Stuffed Keto Wraps------------------- 102

Beef Satay and Peanut Sauce ------------------ 104

Keto Reuben Skillet---------------------------- 107

Mini Meatloaves ------------------------------- 109

Sesame Salmon w. Baby Bok Choy & Mushrooms --- 111

Greek Meatballs Salad--------------------------113

Broccoli Soup with Turmeric --------------------115

Chicken Nuggets ----------------------------------- 117

Low Carb Chicken Philly Cheesesteak ----------- 119

Cauliflower Rice ---------------------------------- 121

Turkey Lettuce Wraps----------------------------122

Low-Carb Zucchini Nachos----------------------124

Chicken Stir Fry ----------------------------------127

Stuffed Bell Peppers-----------------------------129

Dinner Recipes----------------------------------**131**

Chicken Cacciatore -------------------------------- 131

Spicy Eggplant and Pork-------------------------134

Chicken and Sausage Jambalaya----------------137

Cajun Shrimp Skillet -----------------------------139

Bacon Wrapped Chicken Bombs---------------- 141

Rogan Josh--143

Keto Stuffed Meatloaf----------------------------145

Seafood Soup--------------------------------------147

Keto Shrimp Scampi ----------------------------- 151

Lime Pork Chops ---------------------------------153

Keto Cauli Cottage Pie --------------------------155

Slow-Cooker Beef & Broccoli --------------------157

Easy Cashew Chicken----------------------------- 159

Keto Salmon Curry ------------------------------161

Keto Beef Bulgogi ------------------------------- 163

Pan Seared Salmon ------------------------------ 165

Salmon with Pesto Cauliflower Rice ------------ 167

Salmon with Tomato Cream Sauce ------------- 170

Snacks And Desserts ------------------------------ 173

Vegan Coconut Macaroons ----------------------173

Keto Mocha Mousse -----------------------------175

Easy Orange Cake Balls --------------------------177

Cacao Butter Keto Blondies-------------------- 179

Berry Bomb Pops -------------------------------- 182

Pecan Ice Cream -------------------------------- 185

Chocolate With Berries And Cream------------- 187

Coconut Raspberry Slice ----------------------- 190

Chia Seed Pudding------------------------------- 193

Matcha Skillet Souffle -------------------------- 195

Keto Flan --- 197

Bacon Asparagus Bites --------------------------199

Parmesan Crisps--------------------------------201

Keto Popcorn----------------------------------- 203

Smoked Salmon and Goat Cheese Bites ------- 205

Zucchini Nacho Chips-------------------------- 207

Chocolate Chip Granola Bars------------------ 209

Tropical Smoothie ----------------------------- 211

Asparagus Fries--------------------------------213

Savory Spiced Pecans --------------------------216

Chia Seed Crackers ----------------------------218

Bacon and Brussels Sprout Skewers----------- 220

Cheesy Bacon Stuffed Mini Peppers----------- 222

Keto Meal Plan for 90 Days------------------224

Week 1 --------------------------------------- 224

Week 2--------------------------------------- 226

Week 3--------------------------------------- 228

Week 4--------------------------------------- 230

Week 5--------------------------------------- 232

Bonus Meal Plan If You Are Hooked To The Keto Diet -- 234

Week 5 Continued ------------------------------ 234

Week 6 -- 236

Week 7 -- 238

Week 8 -- 240

Week 9 -- 243

Week 10 --- 245

Week 11 --- 247

Week 12 --- 249

Week 13 --- 251

Conclusion ------------------------------------- **254**

About The Author

For most of my life, I did not have to worry too much about my weight; I was not the fittest person but I was also not overweight, which was good enough for me. However, after I gave birth to my lovely son, things changed; I gained quite a bit of weight and I did not exactly like what I saw. I was not as confident as I once was and I was very conscious of how I looked and how the clothes I wore made me look. Once my son turned one and was not breastfeeding as much, I started researching for ways to lose weight.

In my quest to lose weight, I have tried quite a bit of different things from the ketogenic diet and intermittent fasting to smoothie cleanses. Since all these have worked for me, I have incorporated them into my lifestyle and I must say, so far I like what I see.

I understand how difficult losing weight can be and to make it easier for you, I write books on what has worked for me and how you can lose weight to achieve your desired body.

I have still not achieved my dream body but I am happy with the progress so far and that is good enough because life is not perfect and I am okay with good enough.

The Basics: Ketogenic Diet For Beginners

If this is your first encounter (or one of your first encounters) with the Ketogenic diet, you perhaps are wondering what the diet is all about. That's why in this first part of the book, I will dedicate it to covering what the diet is, what it entails, how it works, how it came into being and lots of other beginner stuff.

What Is A Ketogenic Diet?

A Ketogenic diet is simply a way of eating where your meals are supposed to be high in fat, moderate in protein and low in carbohydrates. The main aim of a ketogenic diet is usually to change the metabolism of your body from using carbohydrates as a source of energy to using fats for energy, which is only possible when your body is pushed to the metabolic state of ketosis.

Let me reiterate; you MUST get into ketosis to be considered to be following the Ketogenic diet appropriately.

Now, how is this important?

For you to understand why ketosis and you changing your metabolism is important, you will need to learn how a Ketogenic diet works.

How A Ketogenic Diet Works

When average people like us follow the classic high carb diet (which we do a lot owing to the fact that we follow USDAs guidelines, which place carb rich foods at the bottom of the food pyramid), our bodies usually rely heavily on the glucose produced from the breakdown of carbohydrates for energy. Upon breakdown of carbohydrates into glucose, the glucose is then absorbed into the bloodstream for transportation to different parts of the body. The increasing blood glucose concentrations signal the body to secrete insulin from the beta cells of the pancreas. The role of insulin in this case is to help the cells to take up glucose as the glucose-rich blood flows in different parts of the body. It (insulin) does that by triggering the insulin receptors on different cells, which in turn signals the cells to sort of 'open up' in order to take up glucose, which is then used for energy. Without insulin, the cells cannot open up; the insulin is somewhat like a key that unlocks the lock (insulin receptors).

This system is perfect for our bodies, as it ensures the cells do not starve to death and allows us to utilize the available blood glucose for energy. In fact, glucose is the preferred fuel for the body cells; perhaps because it is easy to break down and use for energy. The other reason is that the body doesn't exactly have any other option but to use the available blood glucose because if it doesn't, high concentration of blood glucose over an extended period are harmful to the cells as the high blood glucose creates an acidic environment. The body therefore has to do everything in its power to remove any excess glucose from the bloodstream. It does that with the help of insulin, which signals the liver to convert any excess glucose to glycogen. This glycogen is then stored in the liver and muscle cells and is used whenever dietary glucose levels are low. Often times, our glycogen stores will fill up (they can only take 2000kcal at a time), something which necessitates insulin to signal the liver to convert the excess glucose to fatty acids and glycerol. These are then transported to different parts of the body where they are stored at triglycerides. Continued accumulation of triglycerides is what ultimately results to weight gain.

This means that weight gain is a factor of excessive carbohydrates intake because glucose, which is produced from the breakdown of carbohydrates, is converted to triglycerides/fat.

The Ketogenic diet seeks to reduce the effect of the carbohydrates significantly by lowering the amount of carbs allowed significantly. For instance, you can only take less than 50g of carbs daily and as low as 20g (don't eliminate-just reduce). The goal is to lower carb intake and pair that with increased fat intake and intake of a moderate amount of proteins, something that forces the body to start relying on fats for energy.

So how exactly does this happen?

When you reduce your carb intake, the body's supply of blood glucose is reduced. This means the amount of insulin that the pancreas secretes also reduces significantly, as insulin is produced in depending on the concentrations of glucose in the bloodstream. As a result, the body is no longer in a state where it is constantly storing fat. The reverse actually happens. To be more specific, reducing your carb intake makes the body to use up its dietary glucose, which is accompanied by reduced insulin levels. The cells continues using up this glucose until it gets to the base level, something accompanied by reduced insulin levels as well. When the body detects a reduction in insulin levels, the pancreas, through its alpha cells, secrete glucagon, a hormone whose role is to signal the liver to convert the available glycogen to glucose where it is used for energy, just like dietary glucose. Since the glycogen stores are limited, the available supplies diminish fast, which prompts the body to look for an alternative source of energy. With the help of the human growth hormone, cortisol and catecholamines, your body is forced to start releasing the triglycerides from the fat stores around the body where they are transported to the liver for breakdown to fatty acids and glycerol. Some body cells have the capacity to utilize fatty acids but some can't. Since they still need energy, the body goes through a series of processes that entail breaking down fatty acids into ketone bodies in a process known as ketosis. Ketones are energy molecules, just like glucose. The good thing about them is that just like glucose, ketones can be used by over 70% of all cells in the body, including brain cells (because they can cross the blood brain barrier). Your goal should be to get the blood ketone concentration to **1.5 – 3** mmol/L. This is where derive the most benefits from following the Ketogenic diet.

So why is the change of metabolism important to you?

Well, it is important because the unique benefits of a keto diet come when your body is using ketones as its main source of energy.

In short, the metabolic state of ketosis is what is responsible for the benefits of a ketogenic diet and is what you should aim for when following a ketogenic diet.

The question now is; how will you know that you are in a metabolic state of ketosis?

Signs Of Being In A State Of Ketosis

1. *Bad breath* – One of the signs of reaching full ketosis is bad breath. So watch out for a fruity smell, which is caused by the elevated level of the ketone acetone in your body.

2. *Short-term fatigue* – When your body transitions from using glucose to using fat, it usually undergoes a difficult time because it is caught up in a situation where it can't access glucose for energy and it is not in a level where it can produce enough ketones to provide it with the energy it needs. So another sign that will show you have reached ketosis is a short-term fatigue that comes from the lack of energy.

3. *Loss of appetite* – Another sign that you are in a state of ketosis is the loss of appetite. When you shift from using glucose to using fats as energy, your body starts to

regulate the hormones that trigger your brain and let you know that you are hungry. This reduces your appetite completely.

4. *Increased digestive problems* – When you start following a ketogenic diet, your diet automatically changes as you start eating foods that you didn't always eat. This usually leads to you having digestive problems like diarrhoea and constipation, which signal that you are in ketosis.

5. *Muscle cramps* – When you get into ketosis, one of the signs that you will get is a muscle cramp. This sign is brought by electrolyte imbalances and dehydration that occurs when you reduce your intake of carbohydrate drastically.

Is Keto Diet For Everyone?

The answer is no. Before you can get started on a keto diet, you need to first visit your doctor and get a health screen that will help you determine if keto diet is for you. This is because there are a couple of conditions that don't allow you to adopt a keto diet.

Here are the conditions where the keto diet is not appropriate for you;

- When you have blood sugar issues like diabetes or hypoglycaemia

- If you are suffering or recovering from an eating disorder

- If you are pregnant

- If you are under any medication

Now that you know what a ketogenic diet is all about, you must be wondering why you need to try it.

Well, there are numerous reasons why a keto diet is good for you. Check these reasons out in the chapter below.

Why The Ketogenic Diet?

One of the reasons why the ketogenic diet is so popular today is because it is a result driven diet. To prove that is true, go to your Google search now and type, 'keto diet success stories'.

What have you seen? Let me guess, numerous stories and before and after pictures that show just how effective the keto diet is.

Ketogenic diet basically changes people's lives for the better and it does that by exposing you to an array of benefits. These keto benefits is what makes big TV stars like Halle Berry, Le Bron James, Vanessa Hudgens and the Kardashians follow the diet and it's the same reason why you should.

So what are these benefits that show why you need to adopt a keto diet?

Here is an extensive explanation of some the benefits you stand to enjoy when you follow a keto diet.

1. **It helps you lose weight**

The number one reason why people adopt a keto diet is because of its ability to help you lose weight- which is understandable considering that we live in a world where 30% of the world's population is either overweight or obese.

But how exactly does a ketogenic diet help you lose weight?

The weight loss benefit of a keto diet comes from the metabolic state of ketosis. As you saw above, when your body is in ketosis, you no longer use glucose for energy. Your body instead switches to burning its own body fats for energy, which it does each and every day. This process of turning your body into a fat burning machine is what enables you to lose immense weight because it eliminates what made you gain weight in the first place.

That said, there are other benefits of ketosis that also have a positive effect on your weight loss.

One such benefit is how the metabolic state of ketosis puts a stop to the process of weight gain. Let me break it down for you.

When your body reaches ketosis, it stops using glucose as its primary energy source meaning the level of insulin in your body drops. If you remember correctly, insulin is a fat accumulating hormone so when it is limited, the process of fat accumulation, which gains you weight is stopped.

The other way that ketosis helps you lose weight is by balancing the hormones that influence weight loss and weight gain in your body. Such hormones include Leptin, your satiety hormone (this signals you to stop eating) and Ghrelin, the hunger hormone (which tell your body that it is time to eat). In order for you to lose fat, you have to have a good balance between the two hormones and that is what ketosis promotes. With that, you automatically reduce your hunger levels and the need for overeating.

2. **It boosts your brain function**

When you follow a ketogenic diet, your brain normally starts to function better than it did on your normal diet. This is usually caused by the combination of carbohydrate restriction and your brain using ketones for energy, which automatically helps you avoid and eliminate brain deficiencies like lack of focus and brain fog.

But how exactly does the use of ketone boost the function of your brain?

When your brain uses ketones as energy, it gets to balance the two important neurotransmitters, which determine the health of your brain. The two transmitters are Glutamate and GABA (gamma-Amino butyric acid). GABA is the main inhibitory neurotransmitter and its work is to reduce stimulation in your body. Glutamate on the other hand is a primary excitation neurotransmitter, which works as a promoter of stimulation in your body.

A lot of times, when we follow our usual high carb diets, the two neurotransmitters fail to balance and our bodies end up experiencing high levels of glutamate and low levels of GABA, which results to brain fog and lack of focus. The reason why this happens is because your brain uses glutamic acid and glutamate as fuel, which results into a shortage of glutamic acid to be converted as GABA. A keto diet helps rectify that situation by providing your brain with another form of energy called ketones. That enables the two aforementioned neurotransmitters to balance, which automatically boosts the health of your brain and brain functions.

3. **It lowers your risk of getting heart disease**

The other reason why a keto diet is so important and worth a shot is because following it usually lowers your risk of developing cardiovascular diseases.

So how does the diet do that?

The keto diet decreases your chances of developing heart diseases by increasing the levels of HDL cholesterol in your body. But aren't cholesterol bad for your heart? The answer is yes and no.

Let me explain;

There are two types of cholesterol:

- LDL- This type of cholesterol is known as the bad cholesterol and this is because its main work is to carry cholesterol from your liver to the rest of your body.

- HDL- This is the good type of cholesterol and this is because it carries cholesterol away from your body and dumps it in your liver where it is either excreted or reused.

When on your keto diet, your level of HDL is increased and your level of LDL is decreased. This combination is the one that reduces your chances of developing heart disease.

4. **It can help reverse type 2 diabetes**

One study conducted in Indiana University tested the effects of a keto diet on type 2 diabetes. This study used 262 people who were overweight and had type 2 diabetes to test its theory.

The research started by all the participants being told to restrict their carbohydrate intake to less than 30 grams every day and increase their intake of fat and proteins instead. They followed that diet for 10 weeks and after that, they were tested and it was discovered that almost 56.8% of the participants had reduced their intake of diabetes medication from one or two of their tablets or had eliminated a full medication all together.

As the study shows, a keto diet helps you reverse type 2 diabetes, which is normally caused by insulin resistance where your cells can't detect the presence of insulin so they end up not opening up to receive glucose that is delivered to them. A keto diet rectifies that by lowering your body's production of insulin to healthy levels which helps in reversing insulin resistance.

5. **It gives you more energy**

The other benefit of a ketogenic diet that will make you want to adopt it is its ability to provide you with more energy.

Let me explain.

As you now know, your body gets energy from the food that you eat. That said, there is a huge difference between the energy that you get when following a high carb diet and the energy that you get when following a high fat diet like a ketogenic diet.

When you eat your normal high carb diet, the energy that you get is usually short lived and so you need to eat regularly to provide your body with glucose which it can transform into energy. This is usually not easy and that's why when you follow a high carb diet, your energy fluctuates from periods of high energy to periods of low energy.

However, when it comes to a Ketogenic diet, things are usually very different. Here, your body experiences more energy that does not fluctuate.

How?

It is simple; when you are on a keto diet, your body uses fat as energy. Since your body has a lot of fat to burn and it still stores more fats, you get high energy that never runs out.

Those are some of the amazing benefits of a ketogenic diet and its okay you can keep smiling. I mean; you don't get to hear about the best diet in the world every day.

Now that you are wowed, you must be curious how one can start following a keto diet. Well, worry not, as the next chapter is going to teach you how.

Getting Started

The moment that you have been waiting for is finally here. You now get to learn how to start following a keto diet.

Excited? You should be.

Now, a lot of people are from the school of thought that starting a keto diet is a hard thing to do but that can't be any further from the truth. Adopting a keto diet is a simple process.

All you have to do is to follow three easy steps. This chapter is going to focus on highlighting and elaborating for you the three easy steps that you need to take to get started on a keto diet. Check them out below.

Step 1: Know The Right Amount Of Macronutrients To Take

The first step in adopting a keto diet is you knowing the amount of macronutrient you are supposed to take when on the diet.

Why is this important?

In the first chapter, you learnt that the main goal of a keto diet is to make your body reach the metabolic state of ketosis. What you may not have learnt then is that reaching the metabolic state of ketosis is determined by the amount of macronutrients you eat. That's why knowing the right amount of macronutrient to consume is important and it's why it is our first step.

So what is a macronutrient and which is the right amount for you to take?

Macronutrients refer to the three basic components of your diet which your body requires in large amounts. The three macronutrients are fat, carbohydrate and proteins.

So what quantity of each are you supposed to take to reach ketosis?

Generally, you need to consume **75% of your calories from fat, 20% from protein and 5% from fats.**

What this means is that if your daily calorie intake is 2500 per day and you take 3 meals in a day, then each meal that you consume will have 625 calories from fats, 500 calories from proteins and 125 calories from carbs.

That said, the specific amount of calories to take as you will come to realize later on is different for everyone because we all have different health objectives, weight loss objectives, activity levels that we do and different body types.

For instance, if your goal is to build muscles when on a keto diet, you will automatically need more proteins and so you can do 25% protein and reduce the fat to 70%. Likewise, if you want to lose weight on a keto diet, you can lower your carb intake to maybe 3% and add the difference to your fat intake in order for you to get into an even deeper state of ketosis where your fat burning process will be intensified. You could even lower the total amount of calories that you take in a day.

So how can you know your ideal macronutrient ratio?

There are two methods that you can use to know your ideal macronutrient ratio.

1. *Experiment*

In this method, you will need to follow the keto diet for about a week or two and then sit down and analyse the changes that the current macronutrient ratio is giving to you. If they are satisfactory to your needs, maintain them but if they are not, then you can start adjusting them slowly by slowly to suit your needs and desires.

2. *Use a keto calculator*

The second method which is the easier of the two methods is using a macro calculator to know your ideal macronutrient ratio.

What is a macro calculator and why is it so special?

A macro calculator is a calculator that calculates your ideal macronutrient ratios. The reason why it's so special is because it takes your weight, age, height, activity levels and goals into consideration when calculating and this makes it very accurate. To use this method, you need a macro calculator and below are links that will take you to some of the best keto calculators.

http://bit.ly/2U5H5Yy

http://bit.ly/2FtEdM7

Now that you know what amount of macronutrient to take, the next step is for you to learn the correct foods to eat when on a keto diet.

Step 2: Learn What To Eat And What Not To Eat

The second step that you are going to take is learning what to eat and what not to eat when on a keto diet and this is because in keto diet, you don't just eat anything in your disposal. There are specific foods that you need to eat and there are specific foods that you need to avoid if you are to adopt a keto diet and enjoy its benefits.

So what are the foods that you are allowed to eat when on a keto diet?

Keto Friendly Foods

Carbohydrates

When on a keto diet, you will want majority of your carbs to come from vegetables that grow above the ground. The rest of your carbohydrates you can get them from fruits and from nuts and seeds.

- **Raw vegetables to take can include-** Asparagus, celery, okra, eggplant, Brussels sprouts, cucumbers, cauliflower, zucchini, arugula, Bok Choy, lettuce, spinach and bell peppers.

- **Cooked vegetables to take can include-** Zucchini, turnips, spinach, shallots, pumpkin, onion, mushrooms, kale collard green, and cauliflower, broccoli, and artichoke and beet greens.

- **Fruits to take can include-** Cherries, melons and berries like blackberries, cranberries, blueberries, raspberries and strawberries. That said, you should consume them in moderation.

Proteins

The proteins that you should take on a keto diet should all come from healthy sources. Here is a list of proteins to take.

- **Fish-** Mahi-mahi, catfish, cod, halibut, trout, salmon, tuna, mackerel and shellfish like lobster, mussels, crab, clams and oysters..

- **Poultry-** Wild game, turkey, duck, quail and chicken. Always to eat the darker fattier meat.

- **Meat-** Goat, cow, lamb, pork and wild games. They should be organic and grass-fed.

- **Whole Eggs**

Fats

The best fats come from saturated fats, monounsaturated fats, natural occurring trans-fats and polyunsaturated fats.

Here are examples of keto friendly fats.

- **Healthy fat oils-** macadamia nut oil, avocado oil, virgin olive oil, coconut oil, walnut oil, MCT oil and flaxseed oil.

Nuts And Seeds

You are free to eat Pine nuts, peanuts, hazelnuts, walnuts, almonds, macadamia nuts, brazil nuts, flaxseed, chia seeds, almond flour and coconut flour.

- **Dairy Products**

You are allowed to take cheese, mayonnaise, heavy whipping cream and Greek yoghurt.

Those are the types of foods you are allowed to eat when on a keto diet.

Next, let's discuss foods you are not supposed to eat when on a keto diet.

Keto Unfriendly Foods

1. **Processed foods like** candy, juice, soda, flour, rice and any manufactured foods that consist of chemical additives

2. **High carb seeds and oils like** soybean oil, grasp seed oil, corn oil, canola oil and margarine

3. **Low fat milk and dairy like** all low-fat cheese and cow's milk

4. **High sugar fruits like** grapes, apples, oranges, pineapple and bananas.

5. **Legumes like** chickpeas, lentils and beans.

6. **Starchy vegetables like** parsnips, sweet potatoes and potatoes

7. **Sugar products like** maple syrup, honey, chocolate, ice cream, cakes, pastries and table sugar.

8. **Grains like-** corn, cereal, oats, rice, paste, bread and wheat.

Basically, you should avoid any food that is high in carbs as it will kick you out of ketosis.

Step 3: Go Out For Shopping And Kick Start The Diet

The last step to adopting a keto diet is for you to make a shopping list and go out to shop for keto friendly foods.

So how can you execute this step?

The first thing that you will need to do when executing this step is to get rid of every keto unfriendly food in your house and in your office.

So take a big bag, go to your kitchen and slowly start placing every food that is not allowed on a keto diet on that bag. Go to your office and repeat the exercise.

At the end of the whole exercise, you can either throw all the foods away or you can donate them to family, friends or those that are in need of food.

Now that your kitchen is free from keto unfriendly foods, it's time for you to sit down and come up with a shopping list that will restock your kitchen with keto friendly foods.

As you write your shopping list, consult the keto friendly food list that you learnt in the previous step.

Once done, hit the market and use the shopping list to shop. Restock your kitchen and start cooking keto friendly meals that will change your health and well being.

That simple, you ask?

Yes, it's that simple to start a keto diet.

The question now is; how do you cook delicious keto recipes that keep you going?

Below is a 30-day keto meal plan that will present you with keto recipes, which will show you how to cook tasty foods when on a keto diet.

Breakfast Recipes

Keto Rolls

Prep Time: 10 Minutes

Cook Time: 12 Minutes

Total Time: 22 Minutes

Servings: 8-10

Ingredients

Filling

2 teaspoons of cinnamon

3 tablespoons of melted butter

Frosting

1 squeeze of liquid stevia

1 tablespoon of lemon juice

¼ cup of butter, room temperature

2 tablespoons of vanilla extract

4 tablespoons of cream cheese

Dough

2 squeezes of liquid stevia

1 whisked egg

½ teaspoon of cinnamon

3 ounces of cream cheese

1½ cups of mozzarella

1¼ cups of almond flour

Directions

Preheat the oven to about 400 degrees.

In a small bowl, put in cream and mozzarella cheese then microwave the cheese mixture for around a minute; remove it and mix well.

Place the cheese mix into the microwave for one more minute and mix again then put in egg, cinnamon, stevia and almond flour. Stir well to combine.

The mixture might be a little wet but if it very wet and sticking on your fingers, then you can add some more flour. Roll out the dough using a rolling pin then spread onto the batter the butter and drizzle some cinnamon.

Roll up the batter from one end to the other until you get a cylinder shape. With a pizza cutter or knife, slice the rolled dough into pieces and put these pieces on a baking sheet coated with parchment paper.

Bake for about 10-12 minutes at 400 degrees F.

In the meantime, prepare the frosting. In a mixing bowl, put in butter and cream cheese and combine until the mixture is creamy, add in lemon juice and vanilla extract. Combine well until everything is incorporated.

When the rolls are ready, add the frosting on each roll; you can add the frosting on the rolls immediately or after about 5-10 minutes.

Nutritional Information Per serving: 5 grams carbs, 320 calories, 11 grams protein, 29 grams fat

Keto Frittata

Prep Time: 5 Minutes

Cook Time: 35 Minutes

Total Time: 40 Minutes

Servings: 4

Ingredients

Pepper and Salt

5 ounces of shredded cheese

1 cup of heavy whipping cream

8 eggs

8 ounces of fresh spinach

2 tablespoons of butter to be used in frying

5 ounces of diced bacon

Directions

Preheat oven to about 175 degrees Celsius then in a skillet, on medium to high heat, sauté bacon in some butter until it becomes crispy.

Put in spinach and mix until the spinach is wilted. Remove the skillet from heat and put aside.

Whisk together whipping cream and eggs then pour the mixture into a coated baking dish about nine by nine inches.

Add in the cheese, spinach and bacon mixture and put the dish in the oven.

Bake for about 25-30 minutes until golden brown at the top and set in the centre.

Nutritional Information Per serving: 4 grams carbs, 59 grams fat, 661 calories, 27 grams proteins

Chorizo Omelette

Prep time: 0 minutes

Cook Time: 15 minutes

Total Time: 15 minutes

Servings: 2

Ingredients

For the toppings

1 slice of crumbled bacon

1/8 cup of avocado, diced

1 tablespoon of sour cream

For the omelette

Pepper and salt

1/4 cup of shredded cheddar cheese

2 ounces of chorizo

2 tablespoons of heavy whipping cream

2 tablespoons of white onion

1/4 cup of chopped spinach

2 large eggs

For the chorizo

2 1/2 pounds of ground pork, precooked

1/2 cup of water

1/2 cup of red pepper flakes, crushed

1/2 cup of distilled white vinegar

3 teaspoons of dried oregano

1 clove of garlic

Directions

Combine water, red pepper flakes, vinegar, oregano and garlic in a blender then blend until the mixture is smooth.

In a mixing bowl, add in the mixture on top of the pork, cover using a lid and put in a refrigerator all day. Get rid of excess water, which accumulates.

Mix together onion, whipping cream, spinach and eggs in a bowl then add the mix into a pan on low to medium heat.

Turn the omelette to the other side when it is becomes firm; you can cover the pan using a lid if it is not becoming firm.

Drizzle some cheese on the other side and evenly cook the omelette, remove from the heat and put on a plate. Add in the chorizo to the omelette and roll the egg then top with some bacon, diced avocado, more chorizo and sour cream.

Nutritional Information Per serving (½ omelette): 378 calories, 2.5 grams carbohydrates, 32.5 grams fat, 18 grams protein

Blueberry Smoothie

Prep Time: 5 minutes

Cook Time: 0 minutes

Total time: 5 minutes

Servings: 2

Ingredients

½ teaspoon of vanilla extract

1 tablespoon of lemon juice

½ cup of fresh blueberries

14 ounces of coconut milk

Directions

Put all of the ingredients in a blender and blend until the mixture is smooth. Taste then add in lemon juice as you wish.

Nutritional Information Per serving: 10 grams carbs, 4 grams proteins, 43 grams fat, 415 calories

Baked Mini-Frittatas

Prep Time; 15 Minutes

Cook Time: 25 Minutes

Total Time: 40 Minutes

Servings: 6

Ingredients

Black pepper, fresh-ground

1/2 teaspoon of spike seasoning

6 eggs, beaten

3 tablespoons of green onions, sliced thinly

3/4 cup of feta cheese, crumbled

1/2 cup of rinsed and drained well cottage cheese

2 teaspoons of olive oil

12 ounces of washed and sliced mushrooms

Directions

Preheat oven to about 375 degrees F then coat 6 muffin cups or ramekins with some non-stick spray and place cottage cheese into a colander.

Rinse the cheese using some cold water until only curds are left. Leave it to drain as you make the mushrooms.

In a fine colander, wash mushrooms then pat dry using paper towels.

Cut the mushrooms into thick slices.

In a non-stick skillet, on medium to high heat, heat olive oil then cook the mushrooms until they are browned lightly and all the liquid has evaporated, for around 6-8 minutes.

Place the cooked mushrooms at the bottom of the ramekins or muffins cups. Slice thinly the onions and crumble feta cheese then layer the green onions, feta cheese and cottage cheese over the mushrooms.

Whisk the eggs with some black pepper and spike seasoning then divide the egg mix equally among the muffin cups.

Using a fork, stir gently the mixture to ensure that all of the ingredients are coated well with the egg. Bake for around 25 minutes until they are browned light at the top and set. Serve immediately with a scoop of low-fat sour cream.

Nutritional Information Per serving: 144 calories, 3.7 grams carbs, 12 grams proteins, 9.5 grams fat

Breakfast Biscuit Sandwiches

Prep Time: 10 Minutes

Cook Time: 30 Minutes

Total Time: 40 Minutes

Servings: 2-4

Ingredients

For the sandwich

Hot sauce, this is optional

A handful of arugula

6-8 slices of bacon, cooked

4-6 scrambled eggs

For the biscuits

Onion powder, garlic powder, paprika and rosemary

¼ teaspoon of baking powder, this is optional

2-4 tablespoons of butter, sliced into pieces

½ cup of heavy whipping cream

2 eggs

1½ to 2 cups of mozzarella cheese

2 cups of almond flour

Directions

Combine together all of the ingredients in a mixing bowl then make small balls using the batter. Bake the balls for around 20 minutes at 375 degrees, until firm.

To make the sandwich, slice the cooked balls into halves then on one half, place scrambled eggs, topped with arugula and bacon. Put the other half on top and enjoy.

Repeat for the remaining balls.

Nutritional Information Per serving: 1107.5 calories, 53.7 grams carbs, 64.9 grams proteins, 68.2 grams fats

Cauliflower Hash Browns

Prep Time: 10 Minutes

Cook Time: 20 Minutes

Total Time: 30 Minutes

Servings: 4

Ingredients

4 ounces of butter to be used for frying

2 pinches of pepper

1 teaspoon of salt

½ grated yellow onion

3 eggs

15 ounces of cauliflower

Directions

Rinse with some water, trim and grate cauliflower with a grater or food processor.

Put the cauliflower in a bowl then add in the remaining ingredients and combine before putting aside for about 5-10 minutes.

In a skillet, on medium heat, melt some oil or butter then keep the oven on low heat to ensure that the first set of pancakes are still warm as you make the rest.

Put a scoop of the batter in the skillet and flatten it until it measures around 3-4 inches in thickness.

Fry for around 4-5 minutes on every side; regulate the heat to ensure that the pancakes do not burn. Repeat the same for the remaining batter.

Nutritional Information Per serving: 5 grams carbs, 7 grams proteins, 278 calories, 26 grams fats

Keto Breakfast Cheesecake

Prep Time: 20 Minutes

Cook Time: 45 Minutes

Total Time: 1 Hour 5 Minutes

Servings: 24 mini cheesecakes

Ingredients

Toppings

1/4 cup of mixed berries for each cheesecake, frozen and thawed

Filling ingredients

1/2 teaspoon of vanilla extract

1/2 teaspoon of almond extract

3/4 cup of sweetener

6 eggs

8 ounces of cream cheese

16 ounces of cottage cheese

Crust ingredients

4 tablespoons of salted butter

2 tablespoons of sweetener

2 cups of almonds, whole

Directions

Preheat oven to around 350 degrees F.

Pulse almonds in a food processor then add in butter and sweetener.

Pulse until all the ingredients mix well and a course dough forms.

Coat twelve silicone muffin pans using foil or paper liners.

Divide evenly the batter between the muffin pans then press into the bottom part until it forms a crust and bake for about 8 minutes.

In the meantime, mix in a food processor the cream cheese and cottage cheese then pulse until the mixture is smooth.

Put in the extracts and sweetener then combine until well mixed.

Add in eggs and pulse again until it becomes smooth; you might need to scrape down the mixture from the sides of the processor. Share equally the batter between the muffin pans, then bake for around 30-40 minutes until the middle is not wobbly when you shake lightly the muffin pan.

Put aside until cooled completely then put in the refrigerator for about 2 hours and then top with frozen and thawed berries.

Nutritional Information Per serving: 12 grams fats, 152 calories, 6 grams proteins, 3 grams carbs

Bacon Cheeseburger Waffles

Prep Time: 10 Minutes

Cook Time: 20 Minutes

Total Time: 30 Minutes

Servings: 4

Ingredients

Toppings

Pepper and Salt to taste

1.5 ounces of cheddar cheese

4 tablespoons of sugar-free barbecue sauce

4 slices of bacon

4 ounces of ground beef, 70% lean meat and 30% fat

Waffle dough

Pepper and salt to taste

3 tablespoons of parmesan cheese, grated

4 tablespoons of almond flour

¼ teaspoon of onion powder

¼ teaspoon of garlic powder

1 cup (125 g) of cauliflower crumbles

2 large eggs

1.5 ounces of cheddar cheese

Directions

Shred about 3 ounces of cheddar cheese then add in cauliflower crumbles in a bowl and put in a half of the cheddar cheese.

Put into the mixture spices, almond flour, eggs and parmesan cheese then mix and put aside for some time.

Thinly slice the bacon and cook in a skillet on medium to high heat.

After the bacon is cooked partially, put in the beef. Cook until the mixture is well done.

Then put the excess grease from the bacon mixture into the waffle mixture. Set aside the bacon mix.

Use an immersion blender to blend the waffle mix until it becomes a paste then add into the waffle iron half of the mix and cook until it become crispy.

Repeat for the remaining waffle mixture.

As the waffles cook, add sugar free barbecue sauce to the ground beef and bacon mixture in the skillet.

Then proceed to assemble waffles by topping them with half of the left cheddar cheese and half the beef mixture. Repeat this for the remaining waffles, broil for around 1-2 minutes until the cheese has melted then serve right away.

Nutritional Information Per serving: 18.8grams protein, 33.94grams fats, 405.25 Calories, 4.35grams carbs

Blueberry Coconut Porridge

Prep Time: 5 Minutes

Cook Time: 5 Minutes

Total Time: 10 Minutes

Servings: 2

Ingredients

Toppings

1 ounce of coconut, shaved

2 tablespoons of pumpkin seeds

60 grams of blueberries

2 tablespoons of butter

Porridge

1 pinch of salt

10 drops of liquid stevia

1 teaspoon of vanilla extract

1 teaspoon of cinnamon

1/4 cup of coconut flour

1/4 cup of flaxseed, ground

1 cup of almond milk

Directions

Let the almond milk heat up on low heat, put in salt, cinnamon, coconut flour and flax seed then combine well.

Use a whisk to get rid of any clumps.

Then heat the mixture until it slightly bubbles before adding in vanilla extract.

And liquid stevia.

When the almond mixture becomes as thick as you like, switch off the heat and put in the toppings.

Nutritional Information Per serving: 405 Calories, 34 grams fats, 8 grams carbs, 10 grams proteins

Egg-Crust Pizza

Prep Time: 5 Minutes

Cook Time: 15 Minutes

Total Time: 20 Minutes

Servings: 1-2

Ingredients

¼ teaspoon of dried oregano to taste

½ teaspoon of spike seasoning to taste

1 ounce of mozzarella, chopped into small cubes

6 – 8 sliced thinly black olives

6 slices of turkey pepperoni, sliced into half

4-5 thinly sliced small grape tomatoes

2 eggs, beaten well

1-2 teaspoons of olive oil

Directions

Preheat the broiler in an oven then in a small bowl, beat well the eggs. Cut the pepperoni and tomatoes in slices then cut the mozzarella cheese into cubes.

Put some olive oil in a skillet over medium heat then heat the pan for around one minute until it begins to get hot. Add in eggs and season with oregano and spike seasoning then cook for around 2 minutes until the eggs begin to set at the bottom.

Drizzle half of the mozzarella, olives, pepperoni and tomatoes on the eggs followed by another layer of the remaining half of the above ingredients. Ensure that there is a lot of cheese on the top most layer. Cover the skillet using a lid and cook until the cheese begins to melt and the eggs are set, for around 3-4 minutes.

Place the pan under the preheated broiler and cook until the top has browned and the cheese has melted nicely for around 2-3 minutes. Serve immediately.

Nutritional Information Per Serving: 363 Calories, 24.1 grams fats, 20.8 grams carbs, 19.25 grams proteins

Basic Oopsie Rolls

Prep Time: 20 Minutes

Cook Time: 35 Minutes

Total Time: 55 Minutes

Servings: 12 rolls

Ingredients

1/8 teaspoon of salt

1/8 teaspoon of cream of tartar

3 ounces of cream cheese

3 large eggs

Directions

Preheat the oven to about 300 degrees F then separate the egg whites from egg yolks and place both eggs in different bowls. Using an electric mixer, beat well the egg whites, until the mixture is very bubbly, then add in the cream of tartar and mix again until it forms a stiff peak.

In the bowl with the egg yolks, put in 3 ounces of cubed cheese and salt. Mix well until the mixture has doubled in size and is pale yellow. Put in the egg white mixture into the egg yolk mix then fold gently the mixture together.

Spray some oil on the cookie sheet coated with some parchment paper then add dollops of the batter and bake for around 30 minutes.

You will know they are ready when the upper part of the rolls is firm and golden. Leave them to cool for a few minutes on a wire rack. Enjoy with some coffee.

Nutritional Information Per Serving: 45 Calories, 4 grams fats, 0 grams carbs, 2 grams proteins

Cream Cheese Pancake

Prep Time: 5 Minutes

Cook Time: 7 Minutes

Total Time: 12 Minutes

Servings: 1

Ingredients

1/2 to 1 packet of Stevia

1 tablespoon of coconut flour

½ teaspoon of cinnamon

2 eggs

2 ounces of cream cheese

Directions

Combine well all of the ingredients in a bowl until the mixture is smooth then heat a skillet over medium to high heat and add in coconut oil.

Add a scoop of the batter in the heated pan and cook for about 2 minutes on both sides. Repeat the same for the remaining batter. Top the pancakes with sugar free maple syrup.

Nutritional Information Per Serving: 365 Calories, 19 grams fats, 8 grams carbs, 17 grams proteins

Breakfast Roll Ups

Prep Time: 5 Minutes

Cook Time: 15 Minutes

Total Time: 20 Minutes

Servings: 5 roll ups

Ingredients

Non-stick cooking spray

5 patties of cooked breakfast sausage

5 slices of cooked bacon

1.5 cups of cheddar cheese, shredded

Pepper and salt

10 large eggs

Directions

Preheat a skillet on medium to high heat then using a whisk, combine together two of the eggs in a mixing bowl.

After the pan has become hot, lower the heat to medium-low heat then put in the eggs. If you want to, you can utilize some cooking spray.

Season eggs with some pepper and salt.

Cover the eggs and leave them to cook for a couple of minutes or until the eggs are almost cooked.

Drizzle around 1/3 cup of cheese on top of the eggs then place a strip of bacon and divide the sausage into two and place on top.

Roll carefully the egg on top of the fillings. The roll up will almost look like a taquito. If you have a hard time folding over the egg, use a spatula to keep the egg intact until the egg have moulded into a roll up.

Put aside the roll up then repeat the above steps until you have four more roll ups; you should have 5 roll ups in total.

Nutritional Information Per Serving: 412.2 Calories, 31.66 grams fats, 2.26 grams carbs, 28.21 grams proteins

Breakfast Salad

Prep Time: 10 Minutes

Cook Time: 10 Minutes

Total Time: 20 Minutes

Servings: 4

Ingredients

Pumpkin seeds, roasted (optional)

1 sliced avocado

Cilantro and red pepper flakes for garnish

4 eggs

1/3 cup of blueberries

1/4 teaspoon of sea salt and black pepper

1/4 teaspoon of garlic, minced

1 tablespoon of water

1 tablespoon of balsamic vinegar

12 ounces of broccoli Cole slaw salad mix

1 1/2 tablespoon of olive oil (divided)

1/3 cup of red onion, chopped

1 1/3 cup of butternut squash, peeled and chopped

Directions

Peel and slice the vegetables then cut the avocado into slices. Put your squash into a microwave safe dish with one tablespoon of water. Steam the squash in the microwave for around 2½ minutes until tender but not mushy (depending on the microwave power). You can also roast the squash on a baking dish and bake for about 15 to 20 minutes at 425 degrees F.

Remove the squash from the microwave, get rid of the water and put aside. In a skillet on medium to high eat put one tablespoon of oil then add in onions. Sauté for about 2 minutes or until until the onions begin to brown. Put in balsamic vinegar, one tablespoon of water, salt, pepper, garlic and slaw. Combine well in the skillet.

Cover using a lid and cook for around 2-3 minutes on medium heat. The slaw will be a bit tender but not well cooked.

Remove from the pan and put in a bowl. Add in the squash together with 1/3 cup of berries then toss well.

Add in the same pan another ½ tablespoon of oil and add in the eggs. Fry them on medium to high heat.

Cook until the yolk is orange and set and is crispy on the outside, for about 3-4 minutes depending on the way you want the yolk to look like. Place a scoop of the slaw on 3-4 plates then put the fried egg over each plate.

Sprinkle on top some salt, pepper, cilantro, pumpkin seeds and red pepper. Place some sliced avocado onto the side.

Nutritional Information Per Serving: 235 Calories, 15.3 grams fats, 13.5 grams carbs, 9.2 grams proteins

Brie & Apple Crepes

Prep Time: 5 Minutes

Cook Time: 15 Minutes

Total Time: 20 Minutes

Servings: 4

Ingredients

Toppings

Mint leaves, fresh (for garnish)

4 ounces of brie cheese at room temperature

1 sweet apple, small

1/4 teaspoon of cinnamon

1 tablespoon of unsalted butter

2 ounces of pecans, chopped

Crepe Batter

1/4 teaspoon of sea salt

1/2 teaspoon of baking soda

4 large eggs

4 ounces of cream cheese

Directions

Place the ingredients for making the batter in a blender and blend until the mixture is smooth then heat some butter in a pan over medium heat.

Scoop the batter in to the pan and swirl the mixture round until the batter becomes thin and is evenly spread on the pan.

Let the batter cook until the upper part becomes dry, for around 2-3 minutes then gently flip the other side using a spatula and cook for another 2-3 minutes.

Repeat the same until the batter is finished and you have made about 12 crepes.

Place them over each other on a platter as you make the fillings. Place one tablespoon of butter in a skillet then toast chopped pecans until they are fragrant but not very browned. Drizzle with some cinnamon and combine well then remove from the pan and place on a plate. Leave them to cool for a few minutes.

Thinly slice an apple together with the brie cheese then place the apple slices on one crepe and garnish with the pecans. Repeat this for all of the crepes, until all the fillings are finished. Drizzle some mint on top and enjoy using a knife and fork. If you like, you can also roll them.

Nutritional Information Per Serving (2 bowls): 411 Calories, 37 grams fats, 6 grams carbs, 14 grams proteins

Avocado Egg Bowls

Prep Time: 5 Minutes

Cook Time: 15 Minutes

Total Time: 20 Minutes

Servings: 1

Ingredients

Pinch of black pepper and salt

3 rashers of bacon, sliced into small sizes

3 large eggs, free range

1 tablespoon of butter, salted

1 halved avocado, the stone removed

Directions

Begin by scooping the avocado flesh making sure to leave a half inch round the avocado then put a large skillet over low heat and add unsalted butter. As the butter melts, whisk the eggs and sprinkle in some pepper and salt.

Put bacon into the skillet and leave them to fry for some minutes before adding the whisked eggs to fry onto the other side of the pan.

Regularly stir the eggs for them to scramble. The bacon and eggs will be ready by about 5 minutes after adding the eggs on to the pan.

If the eggs are ready before the bacon, remove them from the pan and put in a bowl. Add into the bowl the bacon and mix well with the scrambled eggs then scoop the mixture into the avocado bowls and enjoy.

Nutritional Information Per Serving: 500 Calories, 40 grams fats, 11 grams carbs, 25 grams proteins

Keto Breakfast Quiche

Prep Time: 20 Minutes

Cook Time: 45 Minutes

Total Time: 1 Hour 5 Minutes

Servings: 10 slices

Ingredients

Crust

1 large egg

1 pinch of sea salt

2 tablespoons of coconut oil

2 cups of almond flour

Filling

1 pound of chicken, ground

1/2 teaspoon of black pepper

1 teaspoon of salt

1 teaspoon of oregano, dried

1 teaspoon of fennel seed

1-2 grated zucchini, medium

1/2 cup of heavy cream

6 large eggs

Directions

Preheat the oven to 350 degrees F then make the quiche crust by mixing together the salt and almond flour in a blender or food processor.

Put into the food processor egg and coconut oil and mix well until the mix makes a ball.

Place the ball in a lightly greased nine inch baking dish and press it then put aside. It is not a must for you to pre bake the crust.

In a pan, lightly cook and brown the chicken then put aside for it to slightly cool.

Crack the eggs in a bowl and whisk them until they are smooth. Then add in spices and cream.

Mix well then put in cooled chicken and zucchini then combine until well mixed.

Pour the mixture into the quiche crust and level it using a spatula then bake for about 30-40 minutes or until the crust is golden brown and the middle is firm.

Top with a scoop of sour cream then serve.

Nutritional Information Per Serving: 311 Calories, 25 grams fats, 4 grams carbs, 18 grams proteins

Sausage Gravy and Biscuit Bake

Prep Time: 10 Minutes

Cook Time: 55 Minutes

Total Time: 1 Hour 5 Minutes

Servings: 6

Ingredients

Sausage gravy

½ cup of half and half

¼ teaspoon of salt, *to taste*

1 teaspoon of black pepper

½ teaspoon of onion powder

1 ½ cups of chicken broth

1 teaspoon of xanthan gum

12 ounces of pork breakfast sausage, ground

Biscuits

2 egg whites, large

2 tablespoons of butter, frozen

½ teaspoon of xanthan gum

1 teaspoon of baking powder

1 cup of almond flour

Directions

In a mixing bowl, combine together xanthan gum, baking powder and almond flour.

Grate the butter and add into the flour mix then mix using a fork until the mixture looks like coarse crumbs and put aside.

In another bowl, mix the egg whites until stiff peaks form and fold gently the egg white mixture into the flour mix using a spatula.

Mix well until well combined then place the mixture in a refrigerator for a few minutes as you make the gravy.

In a pan on medium heat, cook the sausage until brown then remove the cooked sausage and place on a plate lined with paper towel to get rid of the excess oil.

Add about one tablespoon of oil from the cooked sausage into the pan over medium to low heat then drizzle the xanthan gum into pan while constantly stirring. Cook for around one minute, until browned lightly.

Mix in the black pepper, onion powder and chicken stock then let the mixture to simmer for around 5 minutes to allow the gravy to become thick. Taste and season as you wish.

Mix in half and half and let the mixture to continue simmering for an extra 3 minutes, until the gravy is creamy and thick.

Add into the gravy the sausage then turn off the heat. Preheat oven to around 375 degrees F and put the gravy into a casserole pan. Add in the biscuit mix over the gravy in small scoops ensuring that you distribute the mixture as equally as possible. Bake for about 18-20 minutes until the biscuits are browned and baked and the mixture is bubbly and hot.

Nutritional Information Per Serving: 374.67 Calories, 33.21 grams fats, 4.75 grams carbs, 14.48 grams proteins

Pumpkin Spice Latte

Prep Time: 10 Minutes

Cook Time: 5 Minutes

Total Time: 15 Minutes

Servings: 1

Ingredients

1/2 cup of almond milk

1 pinch of sea salt

1/2 teaspoon of cinnamon

1/4 teaspoon of pumpkin pie spice

2 tablespoons of heavy cream

2 tablespoons of pumpkin puree

2 tablespoons of erytritol

1 shot of espresso

1 tablespoon of butter

Directions

Brown some butter in a pan over low heat then mix the espresso and erytritol in a blender.

Let the mixture combine well while mixing lightly using a whisk. Add into the blender a pinch of salt, cinnamon, pumpkin spice, cream, browned butter and pumpkin puree and blend until the mixture combines.

Add in almond milk since you used espresso to slightly thin out the mixture. Blend for around 10 seconds on high speed then pour into a cup and top with a drizzle of cinnamon and whipped cream.

Nutritional Information Per Serving: 235 Calories, 23 grams fats, 5 grams carbs, 1 grams proteins

Crustless Quiche

Prep Time: 10 Minutes

Cook Time: 60 Minutes

Total Time: 1 Hour 10 Minutes

Servings: 4

Ingredients

Pepper *to taste*

1/3 cup (25 g) of shredded Swiss cheese

1 cup (85 g) of shredded Swiss cheese

1 ½ cups of heavy whipping cream

¼ teaspoon of nutmeg

¼ teaspoon of salt

4 large eggs

8 slices of bacon

Directions

Set the instant to the medium setting then cut the bacon into slices and fry them until crispy.

Put them aside on the paper towel. In a bowl combine together pepper, salt, nutmeg, whipping cream and eggs then using some cooking spray, coat the inside part of a six inch cake sheet.

In the cake sheet, add one cup of Swiss cheese then crumble the bacon and add into the sheet. Pour on top of the bacon the egg batter then put a steam rack inside the instant pot and add in a cup of water.

Lower the cake sheet carefully into the Instant pot and put over steam rack.

If you wish, you can cover the cake sheet using some foil. Cover the instant pot and lock it then cook the cake on high pressure for around 25 minutes. When ready, leave it for 10 minutes before opening the instant pot.

Remove cake sheet carefully from the instant pot then using a paper towel, pat off any water on the quiche. Top using the left 1/3 cup of Swiss cheese then put under the broiler for around 5-10 minutes, until the cheese browns.

Run a knife or spatula round the sides of quiche to remove from the cake sheet then flip it out carefully on a plate and flip again on a serving platter.

Nutritional Information Per Serving: 572.5 Calories, 52.54 grams fats, 3.46 grams carbs, 22.03 grams proteins

Coconut Cream With Berries

Prep Time: 0 Minutes

Cook Time: 5 Minutes

Total Time: 5 Minutes

Servings: 1

Ingredients

1 pinch of vanilla extract

2 ounces of strawberries, fresh

½ cup of coconut cream

Directions

Combine vanilla extract and coconut cream in a blender then blend until smooth. Top with the fresh strawberries.

Nutritional Information Per Serving: 415 Calories, 42 grams fats, 9 grams carbs, 5 grams proteins

Lunch Recipes

Eggplant and Beef Casserole

Prep Time: 25 Minutes

Cook Time: 30 Minutes

Total Time: 55 Minutes

Servings: 6

Ingredients

Sesame seeds for garnish

Fresh parsley, chopped for garnish

Salt and freshly ground black pepper

1/2 400gram can of tomato sauce

1 pound (450 g) of ground beef

10 white and diced button mushrooms

4 slices of diced bacon

1 diced onion

4 tablespoons (60 ml) of avocado oil, for cooking

2 eggplants

Directions

Preheat the oven to 350 degrees F then cut the eggplants horizontally into thin slices; make sure that you have about 15-16 slices.

Drizzle some salt on the eggplant and put aside in the colander. Put two tablespoons of oil in a skillet then add in mushrooms, bacon and onions. Cook until the bacon is well done.

Put in the beef and cook for a few more minutes, until the beef has slightly browned then season with some pepper and salt.

Put into the skillet another two tablespoons of oil then using some paper towel, pat dry the eggplant slices and add them into the skillet.

Cook the slices on each side until they become soft. Repeat the above until all of the eggplant slices are cooked.

Grease, using some cooking spray, a baking dish and add in the mixture then bake in the oven for about 20-25 minutes.

Once ready, garnish with some sesame seeds and parsley.

Nutritional Information Per Serving: 425 Calories, 34 grams fats, 14 grams carbs, 18 grams proteins

Lasagne Stuffed Portobello

Prep Time: 10 Minutes

Cook Time: 60 Minutes

Total Time: 1 Hour 10 Minutes

Servings: 4

Ingredients

Parsley, chopped for garnishing

1 cup of shredded whole milk mozzarella cheese

1 cup of sugar free marinara sauce

1 cup of whole milk ricotta cheese

12 ounces of ground meat

4 large Portobello mushrooms

Directions

Pat the mushrooms using a paper towel to get rid of any compost or dirt then remove the stems if any. Use a spoon to get rid of the brown ribs.

Press the ground beef into four patties then press each patty into every mushroom cap, ensuring that you cover the edges and up to the sides.

Scoop ¼ cup of the ricotta cheese into each of the mushroom caps and press the edges ensuring that you leave a hole in the middle for the sauce. Scoop ¼ cup of the marinara sauce into every mushroom placing it over the ricotta cheese.

Drizzle ¼ cup of the mozzarella cheese over every mushroom then bake in the prepared oven for about 40 minutes at 375 degrees. Top with some parsley and serve immediately.

Nutritional Information Per Serving (1 Portobello): 482 Calories, 36 grams fats, 6.5 grams carbs, 28 grams proteins

Taco Bowls with Cauliflower Rice

Prep Time: 10 Minutes

Cook Time: 20 Minutes

Total Time: 30 Minutes

Servings: 4

Ingredients

Cauliflower rice

Salt and Chili powder to taste

2 tablespoons (30 ml) of coconut oil for cooking

1/2 head of cauliflower, 300 grams, processed into rice-like pieces

Taco bowl

Pepper and salt taste

2 tablespoons (30 ml) of avocado oil for cooking

Dash of chili powder, to taste

2 teaspoons of cumin powder

1 teaspoon of grated fresh ginger

1 diced medium bell pepper

6 cherry tomatoes, diced finely

1 finely diced medium onion

3 minced cloves of garlic

1 pound (450 g) of ground beef

Directions

In a pan, heat up two tablespoons of oil and garlic then add in beef and cook until browned lightly. Put in bell pepper, tomatoes and onion then cook until the veggies become soft.

Put in pepper, salt, chilli powder, cumin and ginger then combine well to ensure everything is well incorporated.

To prepare cauliflower rice, fry the cauliflower in some coconut oil in a pan over high heat for about 5 minutes or until they become soft.

Season with some salt and chilli powder. Serve the taco meat on top of the cauliflower.

Nutritional Information Per Serving: 459 Calories, 38 grams fats, 9 grams carbs, 21 grams proteins

Pork Skewers with Chimichurri

Prep Time: 5 Minutes

Cook Time: 15 Minutes

Total Time: 20 Minutes

Servings: 2

Ingredients

Salt and pepper

1 minced garlic clove

1 1/2 tablespoons of fresh lemon juice

1 tablespoon of freshly chopped cilantro

3 tablespoons of freshly chopped parsley

1/4 cup of diced green peppers

1/4 cup of olive oil

1 tablespoon of coconut oil

1/4 teaspoon of paprika

1/4 teaspoon of ground cumin

1/2 pound of pork shoulder, boneless

Directions

Slice the pork into slices of around one inch thick then season the slices with some paprika, cumin, salt and pepper.

Place the slices into skewers then heat up some coconut oil in a large pan.

Fry the pork skewers on every side until the meat is well done and the pork is browned.

Mix all the remaining ingredients in a food processor, ensuring that you blend a couple of times to make the mixture smooth.

Serve the pork with some of the chimichurri spooned on top of them.

Nutritional Information Per Serving: 450 Calories, 36 grams fats, 1.5 grams carbs, 30 grams proteins

Keto Tortang Talong

Prep Time: 10 Minutes

Cook Time: 30 Minutes

Total Time: 40 Minutes

Servings: 3

Ingredients

3 teaspoons of pork rinds, crushed

1/3 cup of cilantro, chopped

2 teaspoons of salt

1 teaspoon of ground paprika

1 teaspoon of ground coriander

1 teaspoon of ground cumin

1 teaspoon of dried oregano

1 diced and seeded, small plum tomato

1 crushed clove of garlic

1 stalk of green onions, sliced thinly

3 large eggs

500 grams of ground beef

3 pieces of Chinese eggplant

4 tablespoons of coconut oil, divided

Directions

Grill or broil the eggplant on high heat until the skin is browned throughout and soft to touch.

Remove from the grill and put aside.

In a mixing bowl, whisk the eggs and put aside.

Put one tablespoon of coconut oil in a pan on medium to high heat then fry the tomato, garlic and scallions until aromatic.

Add in salt, paprika, coriander, cumin and oregano then cook until the oil has been infused with the flavour, is fragrant and paste like.

Put in ground beef and cook for a few more minutes until almost cooked and most of the meat is not pink then remove from pan and put aside.

Make a small cut at the centre of eggplant along the length then push it open to form a pocket.

With a fork, widen and flatten the sides of the eggplant, as you want to make it look like a canoe.

Put another tablespoon of coconut oil in the same pan and lay one eggplant into the pan then scoop 1/3 of the beef mix into pocket.

Scoop 1/3 of the beaten egg and add onto the beef mixture. Make sure you put enough egg mix to cover the beef.

Push back in the centre any of the egg that pours over eggplant then drizzle with some cilantro.

Cover the pan with a lid to ensure the eggs set; you can add more oil as required.

Gently and carefully flip the eggplant onto the other side, ensuring that you keep the beef/egg mixture in the pocket.

Cook for another minute until the eggs are golden and cooked then remove from the pan and put on a plate.

Repeat the above for the remaining eggplants. Once ready, serve the eggplants with more cilantro and pork rinds.

Nutritional Information Per Serving: 712 Calories, 57.14 grams fats, 6.32 grams carbs, 37.55 grams proteins

Cheesy Zucchini Aglio E Olio

Prep Time: 0 Minutes

Cook Time: 15 Minutes

Total Time: 15 Minutes

Servings

Ingredients

Salt and fresh cracked pepper to taste

1/4 cup of asiago cheese, shaved

1/4 cup of parmesan cheese, grated

1 tablespoon of freshly chopped basil

1 tablespoon of red pepper, chopped

1 teaspoon of red pepper flakes

1 tablespoon of garlic, minced

3 tablespoons of salted butter

1 tablespoon of garlic oil

2 cups of zucchini noodles

Directions

In a skillet, on medium heat, melt the salted butter and garlic oil then after the butter melts, add in red pepper, red pepper flakes and garlic.

Fry for one minute, make sure you don't let the butter to become brown.

Add in the noodles and leave them to cook for around 1-2 minutes or until they become hot.

Reduce the heat and add in parmesan and basil then transfer to a bowl. Garnish with the asiago cheese.

Nutritional Information Per Serving: 725 Calories, 58 grams fats, 8 grams carbs, 11 grams proteins

Grilled Turkey Burger

Prep Time: 5 Minutes

Cook Time: 12 Minutes

Total Time: 17 Minutes

Servings: 4

Ingredients

Pepper and salt

1 tablespoon of olive oil

1 clove of garlic, minced

1/4 cup of freshly chopped parsley

1/4 cup of yellow onion, diced

1 large egg whisked

1/2 cup of almond flour

1 pound of ground turkey breast

Directions

Mix together the garlic, parsley, onions, egg, almond flour and turkey then season with some pepper and salt.

Combine to mix well all the ingredients. Make the turkey mix into four equally sized patties and brush some olive oil on both sides of the patties.

Preheat grill to medium to high heat and coat the grates with some oil. Put patties on the preheated grill and cover with a lid and cook for around 5-6 minutes then flip to the other side and cook for 5 more minutes, covered until the patties are well done.

Nutritional Information Per Serving: 340 Calories, 20 grams fats, 2.5 grams carbs, 37 grams proteins

Chicken with Radishes and Spinach

Prep Time: 5 Minutes

Cook Time: 10 Minutes

Total Time: 15 Minutes

Servings: 2

Ingredients

1 tablespoon of salt

2 cups of chopped spinach

6 sliced radishes

2 cloves of minced garlic

1/4 cup (60 ml) of mustard

3 tablespoons (45 ml) of avocado oil, for cooking

2 cubed chicken breasts (400 g)

Directions

Put some oil in a skillet and fry the chicken until it turns brown then put in spinach, radishes, garlic and mustard.

Cook for an extra 5 minutes or until the chicken is ready and the spinach wilts.

Season with some pepper and salt.

Nutritional Information Per Serving: 577 Calories, 41 grams fats, 2 grams carbs, 48 grams proteins

Dill Pickle Soup

Prep Time: 0 Minutes

Cook Time: 15 Minutes

Total Time: 15 Minutes

Servings: 4

Ingredients

½ cup of cheddar cheese, shredded

½ cup of bacon, crumbled

½ teaspoon of xanthan gum

3 tablespoons of olive oil

1 cup of heavy whipping cream

¼ cup of chicken broth

½ cup of pickle juice

90 grams of finely chopped dill pickle

½ chopped small onion

1 chopped stalk of celery

1 teaspoon of dried parsley

1 teaspoon of garlic, minced

1 tablespoon of butter

Directions

In a large pot, heat some garlic and butter then add in pickles, onions, celery and parsley.

Add in heavy cream, chicken broth and pickle juice then let the mixture boil.

In another small bowl, stir together xanthan gum and olive oil and pour the mixture immediately into the pot.

Frequently stir the mixture until the mixture becomes thick then add in cheddar cheese and bacon before serving.

Nutritional Information Per Serving: 517.5 Calories, 49.83 grams fats, 3.94 grams carbs, 14.09 grams proteins

Caramelized Onion Croquettes Stuffed with Goat Cheese

Prep Time: 10 Minutes

Cook Time: 45 Minutes

Total Time: 55 Minutes

Servings: 4

Ingredients

1/2 teaspoon of cinnamon

1 teaspoon of garlic powder

1 teaspoon of onion powder

8 ounces of herbed goat cheese

1 pound of ground pork

1 pound of ground beef

1 onion

Water

3 teaspoons of whiskey

1 tablespoon of bacon grease

Directions

Preheat the oven to about 400 degrees.

Meanwhile, caramelize the onions.

Place some bacon grease in a skillet over medium to low heat then slice the onion into two and cut again lengthwise to get ¼ inch cuts.

Put the onions into the skillet once hot and leave them to cook for a couple of minutes then with a spoon, break the onions pieces apart the ones that are stuck together.

Stir the onions after a couple of minutes for around 20 minutes.

Whenever you notice the onions sticking to the skillet, put in a teaspoon of the whiskey and combine. Change this with one tablespoon of water until the whiskey is done and now use only water as required.

The onions will be ready when they are brown, sweet and soft. Once ready, cut the onions into very small pieces then in a mixing bowl, mix together all of the ingredients apart from the goat cheese.

Make about 8 five ounce balls using the mixture and with your fingers, make a little hole at the centre of each ball.

Add about one ounce of the goat cheese into the created hole of each of the balls. Make sure the holes are big enough to easily put in the goat cheese. Cover the left space with the remaining burger mix and flatten it; ensure that you smooth all of the seams to avoid the goat cheese bubbling up and out of the hole. Cook for about 30 minutes in the preheated oven then once 400 degrees is reached, broil the balls for another 5 minutes.

Nutritional Information Per Serving: 700 Calories, 48 grams fats, 8 grams carbs, 63 grams proteins

Coleslaw-Stuffed Keto Wraps

Prep Time: 30 Minutes

Cook Time: 0 Minutes

Total Time: 30 Minutes

Servings: 4

Ingredients

Coleslaw

¼ Teaspoon of sea salt, ground finely

2 teaspoons of apple cider vinegar

¾ cup of mayonnaise

½ cup of green onions, diced

3 cups (270 grams) of thinly sliced red cabbage

Wraps and additional filling

Toothpicks, for holding the wraps together

1/3 cup (25 grams) of packed alfalfa sprouts

1 pound (455 grams) of ground chicken, cooked and chilled

16 collard leaves, stems removed

Directions

In a bowl, mix well the coleslaw ingredients using a spoon until combined well.

When the stems are removed from the collard, they will have one strip missing from one side of the collard to around the centre of the leaf.

Put one collard on your working surface then scoop the coleslaw mixture and place on the furthest side of the collard where the stems have not been removed.

Add another scoop of the cooked chicken and top with some sprouts then start rolling the collard from one side to the other making sure to tuck the sides in to avoid your filling from spilling out.

Once you have rolled the collard, insert about one or two toothpicks into the leaf to hold everything together.

Repeat the above for the remaining collard leaves and the filling; you can then divide the wraps into four servings that are 4 wraps for each serving.

Nutritional Information Per Serving: 609 Calories, 50 grams fats, 6.2 grams carbs, 32.7 grams proteins

Beef Satay and Peanut Sauce

Prep Time: 30 Minutes

Cook Time: 10 Minutes

Total Time: 40 Minutes

Servings: 4

Ingredients

Beef Satay & Marinade

1/2 teaspoon of coriander, ground

2 tablespoons of honey

2 tablespoons of Tamari Soy Sauce

2 tablespoons of Fish Sauce

1 pound of flank steak

Thai Peanut Sauce

1/2 teaspoon of Thai Red Curry Paste

1 tablespoon of honey

1-2 teaspoons of Chile garlic sauce

1/3 cup of canned full fat coconut milk

1/4 cup of peanut butter, smooth

Extras

Foil

Bamboo skewers soaked in water for several hours

1 tablespoon of olive oil to oil meat before grilling

Directions

Make the beef satay by cutting the steak into 1 1/2inch slices ensuring that the grain of meat is going lengthwise across strips.

Put the meat into the skewers making sure that you leave a long handle to enable you to hold as you eat the meat.

In a baking dish, combine well honey, soy sauce, fish sauce and the beef then mix well to ensure that the beef is well coated.

Drizzle some coriander on the meat and rub it in then leave the meat to marinate for around 15-20 minutes.

In the meant time, shake well the coconut milk and preheat the grill.

To make the peanut sauce, warm the peanut butter in a small bowl in a microwave; warm for a couple of seconds then add in red curry paste, honey and garlic sauce.

Using a whisk, slowly mix in the coconut milk to the mixture stirring frequently as you add it in.

Add around one tablespoon of olive oil on top of the beef and rub it in to ensure the beef is well coated.

Fold some foil in half and place under the skewer handles as you cook the meat on grill.

Remove meat from marinade and lay them on the grill ensuring that you put a foil under the skewer handles.

Grill both sides of the beef until well-cooked then serve with the peanut butter sauce or any salad.

Nutritional Information Per Serving: 373 Calories, 27 grams fats, 4 grams carbs, 28 grams proteins

Keto Reuben Skillet

Prep Time: 5 Minutes

Cook Time: 10 Minutes

Total Time: 15 Minutes

Servings: 2

Ingredients

1 dill pickle

4 ounces of Swiss cheese

½ cup of mayonnaise

1 tablespoon of Dijon mustard

9 ounces of drained sauerkraut

10 ounces of corned beef

2 tablespoons of butter

Directions

Put some butter in a skillet on medium to low heat.

Put in beef and carefully fry it then dry the sauerkraut.

Remove as much liquid from it and place evenly in a skillet.

Put some scoops of mustard in the skillet with the sauerkraut then put in Swiss cheese and cook until the cheese begins to melt.

Cover the pan to make the mixture to cook faster.

Serve with more mustard and dill pickles.

Nutritional Information Per Serving: 1104 Calories, 93 grams fats, 3 grams carbs, 58 grams proteins

Mini Meatloaves

Prep Time: 0 Minutes

Cook Time: 35 Minutes

Total Time: 35 Minutes

Servings: Makes 12 Mini Meatloaves

Ingredients

1 1/2 tablespoons of Dijon mustard

3 cloves of peeled and minced garlic

1 teaspoon of dry thyme

2 loosely packed cups of finely chopped spinach

1/2 cup of carrots, grated

2 cups of finely chopped mushrooms

1 peeled and finely chopped medium onion

2 large pastured eggs

1 teaspoon of ground black pepper

1 1/2 teaspoon of sea salt

2 pounds of grass-fed pork

Directions

Preheat the oven to around 350 degrees then in a mixing bowl, mix together all the ingredients.

With clean hands, combine well the ingredients until everything is blended together.

Divide equally the mixture among 12 muffins holes then bake for about 25-30 minutes until the meat is well done.

Serve warm with salad or cauliflower rice then place the left overs in a fridge; this can remain fresh up to 5 days.

Nutritional Information Per Serving: 135 Calories, 3.5 grams fats, 3.1 grams carbs, 21.8 grams proteins

Sesame Salmon w. Baby Bok Choy & Mushrooms

Prep Time: 1Hour 20 Minutes

Cook Time: 20 Minutes

Total Time: 1 Hour 40 Minutes

Servings: 4

Ingredients

Main Dish

1 green onion

1 tablespoon of toasted sesame seeds

4 baby bok choy

8 ounces of baby bella mushrooms

4 4-6 ounces of salmon fillet

Marinade

1/2 teaspoon of black pepper

1/2 teaspoon of salt

1/2 lemon juice

1 teaspoon of grated ginger

1 tablespoon of Coconut Aminos

1 teaspoon of sesame oil

1 tablespoon of olive oil

Directions

Combine together all of the ingredients for making the marinade then sprinkle a half of the marinade mixture over the salmon then mix to coat well the salmon.

Cover and put the salmon in the refrigerator for about an hour for it marinate.

Preheat the oven to about 400 degrees then prepare the veggies by trimming rough ends from bok choy and slicing them in to 2.

Cut mushrooms into 1/2 inch slices and sprinkle the left marinade on top of the veggies.

Lay the veggies and salmon on top of a coated baking dish and bake for around 20 minutes or until the salmon is cooked well.

Top the salmon and veggies with sesame seeds and green onions.

Nutritional Information Per Serving: 284 Calories, 12.9 grams fats, 18.2 grams carbs, 28 grams proteins

Greek Meatballs Salad

Prep Time: 10 Minutes

Cook Time: 20 Minutes

Total Time: 30 Minutes

Servings: 4

Ingredients

For the salad

1/4 cup of chopped flat leaf parsley

1 lemon, sliced into wedges

A few lettuce leaves for serving

1 tomato, sliced into wedges

For the meatballs

4 tablespoons (60 ml) olive oil

Pepper and Salt

2 cloves of peeled and minced garlic

A large handful of finely chopped mint, about ¼ cup

2 teaspoons 2 grams of dried oregano

1 pound 450 grams of ground lamb

Directions

Preheat the oven to about 350 degrees F then in a mixing bowl, mix together pepper, salt, garlic, mint, dried oregano and lamb.

Using your hands, make small balls from the lamb mixture.

Put some olive oil in a skillet and sauté the meatballs in portions until they turn brown.

Remove from the pan and put on a baking tray coated with some parchment paper then bake the meatballs in the oven for around 10 minutes to make sure that the meatballs are well cooked in the middle.

Serve with lettuce and tomato wedges then squeeze some lemon juice from the lemon on top and garnish with parsley.

Nutritional Information Per Serving: 399 Calories, 36 grams fats, 2 grams carbs, 20 grams proteins

Broccoli Soup with Turmeric

Prep Time: 0 Minutes

Cook Time: 1 Hour 10 Minutes

Total Time: 1 Hour 10 Minutes

Servings: 2

Ingredients

1 cup of water

2 small heads of broccoli cut into florets

2 teaspoon of chopped fresh ginger

1 teaspoon of turmeric powder

1 teaspoon of salt

1 can of unsweetened coconut milk

3 cloves of garlic

1 onion

Directions

Put half of coconut milk in a skillet over low heat then add in garlic and onion.

Cook for around 5 minutes, until they become soft. Put in the left coconut milk, water, broccoli florets, ginger, turmeric and salt then let the mixture boil for around one hour while stirring frequently and smashing broccoli florets.

Leave the mix to cool before putting in a processor and processing until smooth.

If utilising a mini processor, blend the mixture in small portions.

Serve with some sesame seeds, fresh greens, roasted almonds and yoghurt.

Nutritional Information Per Serving: 439 Calories, 36 grams fats, 17 grams carbs, 8 grams proteins

Chicken Nuggets

Prep Time: 5 Minutes

Cook Time: 10 Minutes

Total Time: 15 Minutes

Servings: 1

Ingredients

Pepper, salt, pinch of garlic powder

23grams of 40% heavy cream

12grams of European style butter

20grams of olive oil

0.5grams of baking powder

2.5grams of coconut Flour

17grams of cooked and shredded chicken breast

22 grams of egg whites, whipped into stiff peaks

Directions

Cut the chicken into small pieces then in a bowl, mix together the chicken, garlic powder, pepper, salt, baking powder and coconut flour.

Mix to coat well the chicken and ensure that the mixture is dry.

Put in oil into the chicken mix and combine again then fold in egg whites until well mixed.

Melt some butter in a pan then add in the coated chicken pieces in nugget sizes and fry for around one minute.

Flip the chicken pieces and fry the other side for around one minute until cooked well.

Remove the chicken nuggets and place on a plate; you can remove any of the left butter out of the skillet and add over the chicken pieces.

Serve the chicken with some cream diluted with water.

Nutritional Information Per Serving: 296 Calories, 41 grams fats, 2 grams carbs, 9 grams proteins

Low Carb Chicken Philly Cheesesteak

Prep Time: 10 Minutes

Cook Time: 15 Minutes

Total Time: 25 Minutes

Servings: 3

Ingredients

3 slices of provolone cheese

1/2 teaspoon of minced garlic

1/2 cup of bell pepper, diced, fresh or frozen

1/2 cup diced onion, fresh or frozen

2 teaspoon of olive oil, divided

1 dash of ground pepper

1/2 teaspoon of garlic powder

1/2 teaspoon of onion powder

2 tablespoon of Worcestershire sauce

10 ounces of about 2 boneless chicken breasts

Directions

Cut the chicken into very thin cuts then place in a freezer for a few minutes to make it easier in making this recipe.

Put the chicken in a bowl and add in Worcestershire sauce, onion powder, garlic powder and pepper; toss to coat well with the chicken.

In an ovenproof pan, put one teaspoon of olive oil then add in the chicken and cook for around 5 minutes or until they turn brown.

Turn the chicken pieces to the other side and cook for another 2-3 minutes, until brown.

Remove from the pan.

Put the left olive oil in the same pan then add in garlic, pepper and onions.

Cook while stirring constantly for about 2-3 minutes until they are hot and soft.

Reduce the heat and put the chicken pieces back into the pan; stir to combine everything together.

Put the cheese on top and cover with a lid for another 2-3 minutes until the cheese melts. Serve in bowls and enjoy.

Nutritional Information Per Serving: 263 Calories, 13 grams fats, 5 grams carbs, 27 grams proteins

Cauliflower Rice

Prep Time: 15 Minutes

Cook Time: 10 Minutes

Total Time: 25 Minutes

Servings: 4

Ingredients

3/4 cup of heavy cream

1 cup of shredded Asiago cheese

3 cups of cauliflower rice

Directions

In a skillet, over medium to high heat, put two tablespoons of water and cauliflower.

Cover with a lid and cook for about 5 minutes.

Put in cheese and cream and combine until the cheese melts.

Taste to make sure that the cauliflower is ready then remove from the heat and serve immediately, enjoy.

Nutritional Information Per Serving: 250 Calories, 21.8 grams fats, 5.6 grams carbs, 7.1 grams proteins

Turkey Lettuce Wraps

Prep Time: 10 Minutes

Cook Time: 6 Minutes

Total Time: 16 Minutes

Servings: 6

Ingredients

12 Boston lettuce leaves

Pinch of salt

2 teaspoons of red chili paste, roasted

1 tablespoon of rice vinegar

2 tablespoon of lower-sodium soy sauce

3 tablespoons of hoisin sauce

1 (8 oz) can of water chestnuts, sliced, drained and chopped coarsely

4 thinly sliced green onions

⅛ teaspoon of ground ginger

1 clove garlic, minced

1 tablespoon of olive oil

1¼ pound of fat-free ground turkey, lean

Directions

Place around one tablespoon of oil in a pan on medium to high eat then add in ginger, garlic and turkey.

Cook for around 6 minutes or until the turkey turns brown; mix to crumble then remove from the heat.

Mix well chestnuts, onions and the turkey mixture in a bowl then stir well to ensure everything is well incorporated and put aside.

In the meantime, whisk together red chili paste, rice vinegar, soy sauce and hoisin sauce then sprinkle on top of the turkey mix.

Toast to mix well all of the ingredients. Add around ¼ cup of the turkey mix to each of the lettuce leaf and enjoy.

Nutritional Information Per Serving: 162 Calories, 4.3 grams fats, 7.8 grams carbs, 23.5 grams proteins

Low-Carb Zucchini Nachos

Prep Time: 20 Minutes

Cook Time: 20 Minutes

Total Time: 40 Minutes

Servings: 2

Ingredients

Toppings

2 sliced green onions

3 tablespoons of black olives, sliced

1/3 cup (38 g) of dairy-free cheese, shredded

MCT Guacamole

Pinch of vitamin C crystals

1/4 teaspoon of finely ground sea salt

1/2 teaspoon of dried oregano

1 tablespoon of apple cider vinegar

1 tablespoon of MCT oil

2 tablespoons of Collagen Proteins Peptides

1 avocado

Meat

1/4 teaspoon of oregano leaves, dried

1/4 teaspoon of red pepper flakes, crushed

1/4 teaspoon of onion powder

1/4 teaspoon of garlic powder

1/2 teaspoon of ground cumin

1/2 teaspoon of paprika

1/2 teaspoon of finely ground sea salt

1/2 tablespoon of chili powder

1/2 pound (225 g) of regular ground beef

Low-Carb Nacho Chips

2 zucchini, medium sized and sliced into thin rounds

Directions

Coat a platter with some parchment paper then put the zucchini on the paper ensuring that you do not overlap them. You might have to cook all of the zucchini in a couple of rounds.

Put the platter with the zucchini into a microwave and cook them for about 8-10 minutes on around 50% power setting.

You will see that the chips are ready when the middle is a bit golden and the sides curl.

Once ready, remove the chips from the microwave and remove the parchment paper on the platter, flip the chips to the other side and leave them to cool. Repeat this for the left zucchini.

In the meantime, put all of the meat ingredients in a large skillet and cook them on medium heat while stirring frequently until the meat is not pink.

Mix together all of the guacamole ingredients in a mixing bowl then mash them until well mixed.

Put the chips on a plate then top with the green onions, olives, cheese and cooked meat.

Serve with the guacamole.

Nutritional Information Per Serving: 578 Calories, 38.6 grams fats, 16.4 grams carbs, 43.7 grams proteins

Chicken Stir Fry

Prep Time: 10 Minutes

Cook Time: 15 Minutes

Total Time: 25 Minutes

Servings: 2

Ingredients

1 tablespoon of garlic powder

3 tablespoons of oil

1/2 cup of sliced thinly celery

1/2 cup of broccoli, chopped

1 medium chicken breast, cooked and shredded

8 ounces of shirataki spaghetti

Directions

Drain the spaghetti from the liquid then in a pan without oil, fry the spaghetti ensuring that you do so until the bottom part of the pan is entirely dry.

Remove them from the pan and put aside.

Put in some oil into the same pan then add in the veggies and chicken.

Cook until the veggies are cooked to how you like them.

Immediately add in the spaghetti together with the garlic powder then mix to combine well and enjoy.

Nutritional Information Per Serving: 325 Calories, 24 grams fats, 7 grams carbs, 29 grams proteins

Stuffed Bell Peppers

Prep Time: 10 Minutes

Cook Time: 30 Minutes

Total Time: 40 Minutes

Servings: 4

Ingredients

¼ cup of shredded Monterey jack cheese

¼ cup of mozzarella cheese, shredded

¼ cup of pizza sauce

1 teaspoon of seasoning salt

1 ½teaspoons of Italian seasoning

1 tablespoon of parsley

1/2 (14 ½ ounce) can of tomatoes, diced with 1/4 cup of the liquid reserved

1 pound of ground turkey

2 tablespoons of minced green peppers

¼ cup of green onion, finely chopped

3 garlic cloves, minced

⅓ cup of onion, chopped finely

1 tablespoon of extra virgin olive oil

4 green peppers, seeds and tops removed

Directions

Preheat the oven to about 375 degrees then fry the garlic and onion in some olive oil until the onion becomes soft.

Put in green pepper and green onions and fry for five more minutes.

Place the onion mix aside then add into the same pan ground turkey and cook until lightly browned and cooked through.

Return the onion mixture back into the pan together with salt, Italian seasoning, parsley and diced tomatoes.

Combine well and cook the mixture for five more minutes.

Scoop the mixture and add it into the green peppers then add the tomato liquid in a baking sheet.

Put the peppers into the baking sheet and garnish every stuffed pepper with around one tablespoon of the pizza sauce and the cheeses.

Bake for about 20 minutes in the oven until the cheese becomes golden brown.

Nutritional Information Per Serving: 298.7 Calories, 16.3 grams fats, 11.8 grams carbs, 27.9 grams proteins

Dinner Recipes

Chicken Cacciatore

Prep Time: 15 Minutes

Cook Time: 65 Minutes

Total Time: 1 Hour 20 Minutes

Servings: 6

Ingredients

2 tablespoons of each freshly chopped basil and parsley, plus extra for garnishing

1/2 teaspoon of red pepper flakes

Sprigs of fresh thyme

7 ounces (200 grams) of cherry tomatoes

1 can (410 grams) of crushed tomatoes

1/3 cup (80ml) of chicken stock

1/3 cup (80ml) of red wine

1 teaspoon of Italian seasoning

10 ounces (300 grams) of sliced mushrooms

1 thinly sliced medium onion

8 cloves of minced garlic

2 tablespoons of olive oil

Salt and fresh cracked pepper

4 pounds of chicken

Directions

Begin by browning the chicken then season it with some pepper and salt on both sides.

Place oil in an iron pot on medium to low eat.

Put in the chicken and cook it on both sides until browned nicely for around 10-12 minutes.

Remove chicken and place on a plate before putting aside.

Put in mushrooms and sliced onions into the same iron pot then increase the heat to medium high and cook for around 10 minutes or until the mushrooms have lost most of their moisture and the onions are translucent.

Put in garlic and cook for an extra one minute.

Add in wine and scrape any of the browned bits at the bottom of the pan.

Simmer the mixture until the wine reduces by half the amount.

Put in chicken stock and tomatoes then mix in chilli pepper, thyme, parsley, basil and Italian seasoning. Season with some pepper and salt to your liking and let the sauce simmer for 5 more minutes.

Put the chicken back into the pot over the onions and tomatoes then reduce the heat and slightly cover the pot with a lid.

Cook on low heat for about 40-50 minutes, stirring occasionally until the chicken becomes tender and the meat is falling easily from the chicken bone.

Drizzle with fresh thyme, parsley and basil and serve right away on top of pasta.

Nutritional Information Per Serving: 233 Calories, 7 grams fats, 10 grams carbs, 34.7grams proteins

Spicy Eggplant and Pork

Prep Time: 15 Minutes

Cook Time: 15 Minutes

Total Time: 30 Minutes

Servings: 4

Ingredients

Sesame seeds for garnishing

Scallions for garnishing

1/8 teaspoon of xanthan gum

1 pound of ground pork

3 cloves of garlic, minced

1 teaspoon of salt

1/2 tablespoon of brown sugar substitute

1 tablespoon of shaoxing cooking wine

1 1/2 tablespoons of tamari

1/4 cup of beef stock

1 tablespoon of red pepper flakes, crushed

1/4 cup of extra-virgin olive oil

1/4 cup of pork rinds, crushed

1 medium eggplant, cut lengthwise

Directions

Soak the eggplants in some salted water, cover with a lid and leave them to sit for about 10-15 minutes then rinse and drain them.

In the meantime, heat the olive oil in a pan until hot then add in pepper flakes.

Stir them for a few seconds and remove from the heat.

Let them sit for some time then strain.

Reserve about two tablespoons of oil and use the remaining oil to pour on top of the eggplants making sure the pieces are well coated.

Damp slightly the eggplants into pork rinds then make sauce mix by mixing together salt, brown sugar substitute, shaoxing wine, tamari and stock in a mixing bowl. Combine well and put aside.

Put the eggplants in a pan and fry them for a few minutes; remove from the heat and put aside. Put in the reserved oil into the pan and fry garlic until fragrant then add in pork and cook until the pork is not pink.

Return the eggplants back into the pan and add in the sauce mix.

Stir well to combine and cook until the eggplants are soft and the sauce has reduced.

Mix in the xantum gum as required to thicken the sauce.

Top with some sesame seeds and scallions.

Nutritional Information Per Serving: 485 Calories, 39.27 grams fats, 5.31 grams carbs, 23.66 grams proteins

Chicken and Sausage Jambalaya

Prep Time: 30 Minutes

Cook Time: 15 Minutes

Total Time: 45 Minutes

Servings: 4

Ingredients

Salt and pepper

1 tablespoon of dried parsley

1 tablespoon of Tobasco sauce

2 cups of cauliflower grinded into rice-like grains

1 cup of tomatoes, diced

1 tablespoon of paprika

1 tablespoon of garlic, minced

4 3-ounce Andouille sausage links, halved and sliced

1 chopped medium red pepper

1 medium stalk of celery, sliced

1 small yellow onion, chopped

2 tablespoons of Cajun seasoning blend

3 tablespoons of olive oil, divided

8 ounces of chopped boneless chicken thighs

Directions

Preheat oven to about 375 degrees F then coat a baking sheet with some foil.

In a bowl, mix together chicken, one tablespoon of olive oil, pepper and salt then put on the coated baking sheet and drizzle with one tablespoon of Cajun seasoning.

Bake for about 22-25 minutes until well-cooked then put aside for the chicken to cool.

Heat the left oil in a deep pan on medium to high heat then add in onion and cook for around 3-4 minutes.

Mix in red pepper and celery and fry for another 6-8 minutes until soft.

Add in paprika, garlic and sliced sausage then stir well and cook for 2 minutes then add in cauliflower rice and tomatoes.

Cook until the rice is soft, for about 4-5 minutes.

Put in the chicken together with the remaining Cajun seasoning, parsley and tabasco sauce.

Cook until cooked through then serve in bowls and enjoy.

Nutritional Information Per Serving: 415 Calories, 25 grams fats, 10.5grams carbs, 31grams proteins

Cajun Shrimp Skillet

Prep Time: 5 Minutes

Cook Time: 10 Minutes

Total Time: 15 Minutes

Servings: 2

Ingredients

Chopped fresh parsley, for garnishing

1 knob of grated fresh ginger

1 teaspoon of chili pepper flakes, crushed

1 tablespoon of dried garlic

2 tablespoons of Cajun seasoning

1 knob of butter

2 tablespoons of olive oil

Salt and Pepper

1 pound (450g) of large, peeled and deveined shrimp

Directions

In a bowl, put in shrimp and season with some pepper and salt then put in Cajun season and olive oil.

Combine until well coated then in a pan on medium heat, melt some butter.

Put in the shrimp into the pan and drizzle with pepper flakes, ginger and garlic.

Cook for a couple of minutes on each side until it is cooked through and pink.

Put in the pan two tablespoons of water or broth and deglaze the browned bits and spices at the bottom of the pan to coat the shrimp well.

Season with pepper and salt as desired then top with more peppers flakes and parsley.

Serve right away on top of lettuce wraps, broccoli mash or zucchini noodles.

Nutritional Information Per Serving: 131 Calories, 6 grams fats, 2 grams carbs, 16 grams proteins

Bacon Wrapped Chicken Bombs

Prep Time: 5 Minutes

Cook Time: 55 Minutes

Total Time: 1 Hour

Servings: 6

Ingredients

12 slices of bacon

Salt and pepper to taste

½ cup of full-fat ricotta

4 ounces of softened cream cheese

10 ounces of frozen spinach

2 pounds (about 3) boneless, skinless, chicken breasts

Directions

Thaw spinach and drain as much water from it as possible then preheat the oven to about 375 degrees F.

In a bowl, combine ricotta, cream cheese and spinach then season with pepper and salt.

Slice the chicken into two ensuring that the halves are thick enough to make pouches from it.

Gently slice pockets into the end part of each chicken but if you accidentally slice all the way through, it is no big deal, as the bacon will help in fixing this.

Scoop the cheese mix and put into each of the pockets then wrap tightly two slices of the bacon round the chicken pieces.

Make sure to seal any opening or holes that the filling might seep from.

However, do no wrap the bacon so tight round the chicken, as this might make it hard for the chicken to cook through.

In a hot pan, cook the bacon for a few seconds; it is not a must to brown every side of the bacon, as they will still be put in the oven. Put the cooked chicken pieces on a baking dish as you cook the other pieces.

Bake for about 35-45 minutes until chicken is well done and the bacon is crisped well.

Nutritional Information Per Serving: 384.83 Calories, 20.48 grams fats, 2.3 grams carbs, 44.75 grams proteins

Rogan Josh

Prep Time: 1 Hour 10 Minutes

Cook Time: 1 Hour 20 Minutes

Total Time: 2 Hours 30 Minutes

Servings: 1

Ingredients

Sea salt

White pepper

4 grams of fresh, minced cilantro

25 grams of chopped macadamia nuts

20 grams of coconut milk, full fat

200 grams of chicken broth

20 grams of ghee

1 gram of garam masala

1 gram of chili powder

2 grams of fresh, minced ginger root

2 grams of minced fresh garlic, minced

10 grams of onions, cut into small cubes

70 grams of raw lamb, leg meat trimmed of fat

Directions

Mix the last six ingredients and marinate the meat for about one hour or overnight if you like.

Put some ghee in a skillet on medium to high heat and put in the meat together with the ingredients used to marinate the meat then cook until the meat turns brown.

Put in chicken broth into the meat then cover with a lid and reduce the heat to low.

Simmer the mixture for about one hour; you can add water if required.

After the meat becomes soft, remove from the heat and put in macadamia nuts and mayonnaise.

Mix well until combined then season with some pepper and salt, garnish with cilantro.

Nutritional Information Per Serving: 506 Calories, 46 grams fats, 5 grams carbs, 18 grams proteins

Keto Stuffed Meatloaf

Prep Time: 20 Minutes

Cook Time: 1 Hour

Total Time: 1 Hour 20 Minutes

Servings: 8

Ingredients

¼ cup of mushrooms

½ cup of spinach

¼ cup of green onions, chopped

¼ cup of onions, chopped

6 slices of cheddar cheese

500 grams of ground beef

Directions

In a medium bowl, combine cumin, garlic, pepper and salt then in a baking pan coated with some cooking spray, add in half the minced beef.

Make sure to cover the sides and bottom with the beef and leave a hole in the middle for the stuffing.

Place cheese over the beef then add in mushrooms, spinach and onions.

Place the remaining beef over the top to cover mushrooms and spinach.

Bake for about one hour at 350 degrees F.

Nutritional Information Per Serving: 248.63 Calories, 19.56 grams fats, 1.42 grams carbs, 15.8 grams proteins

Seafood Soup

Prep Time: 25 Minutes

Cook Time: 1 Hour

Total Time: 1 Hour 25 Minutes

Servings: 6

Ingredients

Soup

1 lemon

1 lime

8 ounces of mushrooms

1 medium onion

4 cloves of garlic

4 stalks of green onion

4 stalks of celery

3 medium carrots

2 cups of water

1 quart of seafood broth

1/2 cup of coconut cream

1.5 cup of tomato sauce

1/4 cup of coconut oil

8 ounces of shrimp

8 ounces of calamari

10 ounces of wild caught cod

Spices

Fresh parsley

2 teaspoons of oregano

2 teaspoons of basil

3 whole bay leaves

1 teaspoon of dill

1 teaspoon of thyme

2 teaspoons of red pepper flakes

2 teaspoons of pepper

1 tablespoon of salt

Directions

Begin by adding two tablespoons of coconut oil in a pot over medium heat then put in garlic and onion.

Cook until aromatic then add in celery and carrots.

Leave the vegetables to cook until they are soft.

Add in the broth, tomato sauce and water then leave this to boil before lowering the heat.

Let the broth and vegetables to simmer for around 30 minutes before seasoning with pepper and salt.

As the soup boils, peel the shrimp then slice the calamari into pieces of around ½ inch and put them in a mixing bowl with some lemon juice.

The lemon juice helps in avoiding the calamari and shrimp from becoming rubbery if they are cooked for long.

Cut the mushrooms and put into the soup after it has boiled for 30 minutes together with cream.

After the mushrooms cook for around 10 minutes, put in the cod and leave it to cook for another 10 minutes.

Using a spoon, break down the fish inside the pot into smaller chunks making sure to only add the shrimp after confirming that the water is boiling.

Increase the heat, put in shrimp together and leave them to cook for around 3 minutes.

Put in calamari after the 3 minutes into the soup and leave the soup to cook for an extra 2 minutes.

Make sure you do not overcook as the shrimp becomes hard and calamari rubbery.

Switch off the flame and remove pot from heat then put in lime juice.

Make sure you remove the bay leaves.

Serve with fresh parsley and green onions.

Nutritional Information Per Serving: 284 Calories, 14 grams fats, 9 grams carbs, 27 grams proteins

Keto Shrimp Scampi

Prep Time: 20 Minutes

Cook Time: 10 Minutes

Total Time: 30 Minutes

Servings: 2

Ingredients

2 tablespoons of chopped parsley

1 pound of shrimp deveined

Salt and pepper to taste

1/8 teaspoon of red chili flakes

2 tablespoons of lemon juice

1/4 cup of white wine

2 tablespoons of butter

2 summer squash

Directions

Slice the squash into noodles with a spiralizer and place the noodles on paper towels.

Drizzle them with some salt and put aside for about 15-30 minutes.

Pat away the excess moisture from the noodles using the paper towels; make sure the towels are dry.

In a skillet, on medium heat, melt some butter then put in chili flakes, lemon juice and chicken broth.

Let the mixture lightly boil then put in shrimp and boil until the shrimp starts to become pink.

Reduce the heat to low and season with some pepper and salt to your liking.

Put in the noodles and parsley then stir to coat well noodles with the sauce and to evenly distribute the shrimp.

Transfer to a platter and enjoy.

Nutritional Information Per Serving: 366 Calories, 15 grams fats, 7 grams carbs, 49 grams proteins

Lime Pork Chops

Prep Time: 15 Minutes

Cook Time: 3 Hours 30 Minutes

Total Time: 3 Hours 45 Minutes

Servings: 8

Ingredients

3/4 teaspoon of black pepper

3/4 teaspoon of salt

3/4 teaspoon of garlic powder

1/2 teaspoon of ground cumin

5 tablespoons of lime juice

1/2 cup of salsa

3 tablespoons of butter

3.32 pounds of pork sirloin chop- bone in

Directions

Melt some butter in a saucepan over medium to high heat then preheat crockpot as you make the pork chops.

In a mixing bowl, put in all the spices and combine well then put in the chops; make sure to rub in the spice mixture into the pork.

Add in the chops into the sauce pan and cook for about 5 minutes until browned on both sides.

In another mixing bowl, combine lime juice and salsa then when the pork chops are ready, add them in a crock pot.

Put over the pork chops the salsa mixture then cook on high heat for about 3-4 hours until the pork reads about 160 degrees.

Nutritional Information Per Serving: 364 Calories, 17 grams fats, 3 grams carbs, 51 grams proteins

Keto Cauli Cottage Pie

Prep Time: 5 Minutes

Cook Time: 1 Hour 30 Minutes

Total Time: 1 Hour 35 Minutes

Servings: 4

Ingredients

100grams of fried bacon pieces

1/4 cup of tomato puree

1 tablespoon of mixed spice blend

1-2 teaspoons of salt

1 tablespoon of butter

1/2 chopped white onion

500grams of steak mincemeat

For the caulimash

1 tablespoon of herbal salt

1/3 cup of grass-fed butter

1 1/2 - 2 kilograms of fresh cauliflower

Directions

Preheat oven to about 180 degrees Celsius then in a pan over medium heat, sauté onions in the butter until they begin to turn translucent and they are soft.

Put in mincemeat and break it up to ensure the meat does not cluster.

Put in the spices and cook while stirring frequently until the meat becomes brown.

Add in tomato puree and combine well then let the sauce cook for around 10 minutes over medium heat.

Transfer sauce to a baking dish.

Prepare caulimash by cutting cauliflower and getting rid of thick core then place in a pot.

Put in water ensuring that you cover the entire cauliflower then let the mixture boil over medium heat for around 20-25 minutes until the cauliflower is very soft.

Drain the water and season with some salt and butter then put in a blender.

Blend well until very creamy and smooth.

Top the meat with bacon and caulimash then bake for around 30-45 minutes, serve and enjoy.

Nutritional Information Per Serving: 913 Calories, 72.2 grams fats, 37.7 grams carbs, 36.8 grams proteins

Slow-Cooker Beef & Broccoli

Prep Time: 0 Minutes

Cook Time: 6 Hours 10 Minutes

Total Time: 6 Hours 10 Minutes

Servings: 4

Ingredients

1 teaspoon of sesame seeds, for garnishing

1 red bell pepper

1 head broccoli

1/4 - 1/2 teaspoon of red pepper flakes

3 minced garlic cloves

1 teaspoon of ginger, freshly grated

1/2 teaspoon of salt

3 tablespoons of Stevia Blend

1 cup of beef broth

2/3 cup of coconut liquid aminos

2 pounds of flank steak

Directions

Preheat your slow cooker to low.

Then cut the steak into 1 inch pieces.

Into the slow cooker, add in salt, red pepper flakes, garlic cloves, ginger, sweetener, beef broth, aminos and the steak.

Cook for around 5-6 hours on low heat then make the bell pepper and broccoli.

Cut the broccoli into florets and the bell pepper into big 1 inch chunks.

Once the steak is ready, stir well then put in the bell pepper and broccoli.

Cook for about one hour until done then stir again to combine.

Drizzle with some sesame seeds, serve and enjoy.

Nutritional Information Per Serving: 430 Calories, 19 grams fats,4 grams carbs, 54 grams proteins

Easy Cashew Chicken

Prep Time: 15 Minutes

Cook Time: 10 Minutes

Total Time: 25 Minutes

Servings: 3

Ingredients

Salt + Pepper

1/4 medium white onion

1 tablespoon of green onions

1 tablespoon of sesame seeds

1 tablespoon of sesame oil

1 tablespoon of garlic, minced

1/2 tablespoon of chili garlic sauce

1 1/2 tablespoons of liquid aminos

1 tablespoon of rice wine vinegar

1/2 teaspoon of ground ginger

1/2 medium green bell pepper

1/4 cup of raw cashews

2 tablespoons of coconut oil

3 chicken thighs, raw, boneless and skinless

Directions

Heat a skillet on low heat and toast cashews for about 8 minutes until they become aromatic and brown lightly.

Remove from the heat and put aside.

Cut the chicken into 1 inch cuts then slice the pepper and onion into big cuts.

Turn the heat to high and put in some coconut oil.

After the oil has heated up, put in chicken and leave it to cook well for around 5 minutes.

When chicken is done, put in garlic sauce, garlic, onions, pepper and season with some pepper, ginger and salt.

Leave the mixture to cook over high heat for about 2-3 minutes then put in cashews, vinegar and aminos.

Cook the sauce on high heat until the liquid reduces and the mixture becomes thick and sticky.

Ensure that there is no excess amount of liquid in the skillet when done cooking. Serve in small bowls and garnish with sesame seeds then sprinkle with some sesame oil.

Nutritional Information Per Serving: 333.3 Calories, 24 grams fats, 8 grams carbs, 22.6 grams proteins

Keto Salmon Curry

Prep Time: 10 Minutes

Cook Time: 15 Minutes

Total Time: 25 Minutes

Servings: 2

Ingredients

2 tablespoons of chopped basil, for garnishing

Pepper and salt

2 tablespoons of coconut oil

1 pound of raw salmon, diced

2 cups of bone broth

Cream from the top of 1 (14-oz) can of coconut milk

1 teaspoon of garlic powder

1 1/2 tablespoons of curry powder

2 cups of diced green beans

1/2 diced medium onion

Directions

Put the onions in coconut oil in a pan on medium heat then cook the onions until they become translucent.

Put in green beans and fry for a couple of minutes.

Add in broth and let the mixture boil for a few minutes before adding salmon, garlic powder and curry powder.

Stir to combine well then add in coconut cream and leave the mixture to simmer for about 3-5 minutes or until the salmon is ready.

Season with pepper and salt then serve with basil.

Nutritional Information Per Serving: 640 Calories, 44 grams fats, 16 grams carbs, 49 grams proteins

Keto Beef Bulgogi

Prep Time: 15 Minutes

Cook Time: 15 Minutes

Total Time: 30 Minutes

Servings: 5

Ingredients

1 teaspoon of coconut flour

1 teaspoon of salt

1 teaspoon of ground ginger

1 teaspoon of garlic powder

1 tablespoon of apple cider vinegar

2 tablespoon of coconut aminos

3 tablespoons of coconut oil

1pound of skirt steak

Directions

Tenderize the meat using kitchen mallet then cut it into thin slices.

Put in a mixing bowl with apple cider vinegar and coconut aminos then let it marinate for about 10 minutes.

Put in oil in a skillet over medium-low heat then add in the strips once the oil is hot and cook them in portions for about 3-4 minutes for every batch to enable the meat to brown quickly.

After the slices are ready, put them back into the skillet and add in coconut flour before stirring the slices well to coat well.

Put into the skillet coconut aminos and vinegar that was used in marinating the beef then fry for a few minutes until the meat becomes glazed with the sauce.

Serve with cauliflower rice and garnish with ginger, salt and garlic powder.

Nutritional Information Per Serving: 242 Calories, 18 grams fats, 3 grams carbs, 24.9 grams proteins

Pan Seared Salmon

Prep Time: 0 Minutes

Cook Time: 20 Minutes

Total Time: 20 Minutes

Servings: 6

Ingredients

2 tablespoons of Parmesan cheese, grated

2 teaspoons of fresh dill

1 tablespoon of lemon juice

2 tablespoons of capers

1-ounce of cream cheese

1 cup of heavy whipping cream

2 cloves of garlic, minced

3 (6-ounce) of salmon fillets

2 tablespoons of olive oil

Directions

Heat some oil in a large pan on medium to high heat.

After the pan becomes hot, put in salmon and fry for about 5 minutes on every side.

After the salmon is cooked well, put aside as you make the sauce.

Fry some minced garlic in the same skillet until aromatic then put in capers, lemon juice, cream cheese and heavy cream.

Let the mixture to simmer, stirring constantly until the mixture thickens.

After the sauce becomes thick, put in salmon back into the skillet and combine to coat well the salmon.

Lower the heat to medium-low to warm up the salmon for a few minutes. Garnish with parmesan cheese and fresh dill.

Nutritional Information Per Serving: 494.01 Calories, 30.67 grams fats, 2.15 grams carbs, 53.56 grams proteins

Salmon with Pesto Cauliflower Rice

Prep Time: 20 Minutes

Cook Time: 20 Minutes

Total Time: 40 Minutes

Servings: 3

Ingredients

1/2 cup of olive oil

1/2 teaspoon of pink salt

Juice of 1 lemon

1/4 cup of hemp hearts

3 garlic cloves

1 cup of fresh basil leaves, chopped

1 tablespoon of butter

Pinch of salt

1 tablespoon of coconut aminos

1 teaspoon of Red Boat Fish sauce

1 tablespoon of olive oil

3 salmon filets, about 4 ounces each

Directions

Put olive oil, fish sauce and coconut aminos then pat salmon dry using a paper towel and put the salmon in the marinade.

Put the salmon meat side down on marinade then season with some salt.

Let the salmon sit for about 20 minutes.

Heat a pan over medium heat then dice the garlic and add into a processor or blender.

Put in MCT powder, olive oil, salt, lemon juice, hemp hearts and basil then blend to mix all the ingredients.

In a pan, heat the cauliflower to thaw it then proceed to add in a couple of spoonfuls of the sauce that you made and drizzle with salt.

Mix to combine everything then reduce the heat to keep the mixture warm as you make the salmon.

Transfer the rice to a plate.

After the pan has cooled, put in butter and leave it to melt then spread it equally in the pan.

Put in the salmon, the meat side up, and cook for around or 5 minutes until the sides of the salmon look cooked. If the salmon is thick, it will take more time to cook.

Flip and cook the other side of the salmon then add in the remaining marinade.

Cook for around 1-2 minutes.

Transfer to a platter and serve on top of the cauliflower rice.

Nutritional Information Per Serving: 647 Calories, 51 grams fats, 10.1 grams carbs, 33.8 grams proteins

Salmon with Tomato Cream Sauce

Prep Time: 10 Minutes

Cook Time: 15 Minutes

Total Time: 25 Minutes

Servings: 2

Ingredients

Seafood Salmon

2-6 ounce filets of Keta salmon

Bacon and Tomato Cream Sauce

Salt and pepper to taste

1/2 teaspoon of grated lemon zest

10 leaves basil, chiffonade

1 tablespoon of vodka

2 tablespoons of water

1/3 cup of heavy cream

1 tablespoon of tomato paste

1/4 cup of vodka

1 ounce of sliced onion

1 clove of sliced garlic

1 teaspoon of bacon grease

2 slices of diced bacon

Directions

Leave salmon to come to room temperature for about 15 minutes then slice the bacon into cubes.

Put a skillet on medium heat then put in one teaspoon of bacon grease and bacon before mixing to coat the bacon well.

Leave the bacon to cook for around 2 minutes.

In the meantime, cut the garlic and onion into slices, grate lemon zest and chiffonade basil then put the bacon into the skillet.

Stir to cook well the bacon until crisp and browned then remove bacon but leave the fat in the skillet.

Get rid of almost all the fat from the skillet apart from around 2 tablespoons and return skillet back to stove on medium heat.

Salt lightly each of the salmon fillets and put them into the skillet, the skin side up.

Let the salmon cook for around 3-4 minutes undisturbed; this depends on how thick they are. You will notice that the salmon becomes lighter when it is cooked and you will want the salmon colour to change halfway through before you flip them.

Flip to the other side using a spatula and cook for another 3-4 minutes then place on a platter and wrap gently with a foil to keep it warm.

To make the sauce, return skillet back to the stove on medium to low heat then add in garlic and onions.

Stir until the onions become soft for around one and a half minutes then remove skillet from heat.

Add some vodka in the skillet and place the pan back to the heat, scraping up the bits from bottom side of pan.

Leave vodka to evaporate by half.

Add in tomato paste and mix it round the cooked onions to make it warm and help in breaking it.

Put in water and heavy cream, mixing to combine then let the mixture gently simmer for about one minute to make it thick.

Add in lemon zest, one tablespoon of vodka and bacon, then mix well until the smell of alcohol has reduced.

Put in basil then season with some pepper and salt before turning off the heat.

Place salmon on a plate then serve with half the sauce and top with more basil if you like

Nutritional Information Per Serving: 431 Calories, 19 grams fats, 6 grams carbs, 38 grams proteins

Snacks And Desserts

Vegan Coconut Macaroons

Prep Time: 5 Minutes

Cook Time: 18 Minutes

Total Time: 23 Minutes

Servings: 24 macaroons

Ingredients

1/2 cup of vegan melted dark chocolate, for dipping

Pinch of salt

1/2 teaspoon of almond extract

1 teaspoon of vanilla extract

1/2 cup of aquafaba

1/2 cup of monk fruit sweetener

1/2 cup of almond flour

2.5 cups of unsweetened coconut, shredded and divided

Directions

Preheat the oven to about 350 degrees F then coat a baking sheet with some parchment paper.

Put one cup of the unsweetened coconut in the oven and toast for around 8-10 minutes.

In a mixing bowl, add in all of the ingredients together with the coconut and combine well.

Put about one scoop of the batter on a baking sheet then bake for about 18-20 minutes.

Melt about ½ a cup of chocolate then after the cookies are cooked and have cooled, dip the bottom part of the cookies in the melted chocolate.

Put the cookies on the parchment paper and place in a fridge for the chocolate to set for around 5-10 minutes.

If the cookies are not being dipped in chocolate, then you do not have to refrigerate them.

Serve with non-dairy milk.

Nutritional Information Per Serving: 120 Calories, 7 grams fats, 15 grams carbs, 1 gram proteins

Keto Mocha Mousse

Prep Time: 2 Hours 50 Minutes

Cook Time: 0 Minutes

Total Time: 2 Hours 50 Minutes

Servings: 4

Ingredients

For the cream cheese mixture

3 teaspoons of instant coffee powder

1/4 cup of unsweetened cocoa powder

1/3 cup of granulated stevia erythritol blend

1 ½ teaspoons of vanilla extract

2 tablespoons of softened butter

3 tablespoons of sour cream

8 ounces of softened cream cheese

For the whipped cream mixture

½ teaspoon of vanilla extract

1 ½ teaspoons of granulated stevia erythritol blend

2/3 cup of heavy whipping cream

Directions

Combine butter, sour cream and cream cheese in a mixing bowl using a hand mixer and then mix until it becomes smooth.

Add in coffee powder, cocoa powder, sweetener and vanilla extract into the bowl and blend again until all the ingredients have been well incorporated, put aside.

In another bowl, whisk the whipping cream until a soft peak forms then put in vanilla extract and sweetener.

Whisk again until a stiff peak forms.

Fold in 1/3 of the cream mixture into the cream cheese mixture to help in lightening the cheese mixture, making sure you do not deflate bubbles.

Add in the left 2/3 cream mix and mix well until the cream is equally incorporated.

Place the mouse into serving bowls and place in refrigerator until it sets for around 2 ½ hours before you serve it.

Nutritional Information Per Serving: 421.75 Calories, 41.94 grams fats, 6.57 grams carbs, 6.03 grams proteins

Easy Orange Cake Balls

Prep Time: 0 Minutes

Cook Time: 15 Minutes

Total Time: 15 Minutes

Servings: 15 balls

Ingredients

Pinch of pink salt

1/2 teaspoon of vanilla

35 drops of sweet leaf vanilla crème stevia to taste

1/4 cup of orange juice

Zest of 2 navel oranges

1/3 cup of coconut flour plus more for rolling

Heaping 2/3 cup of almond butter

Directions

Mix all of the ingredients in a medium bowl.

If the mixture is too dry, add in some orange juice or sprinkle with avocado.

If the mixture is too wet, put in a drizzle of coconut flour.

Take small scoops of the batter and create into balls using your hands to make the balls smooth and into a rounded shape.

Roll lightly each of the balls in some coconut flour then place the balls in the fridge for about 10 minutes to firm them up.

Enjoy

Nutritional Information Per Serving (One ball): 92 Calories, 7 grams fats, 4 grams carbs, 3 grams proteins

Cacao Butter Keto Blondies

Prep Time: 15 Minutes

Cook Time: 20 Minutes

Total Time: 35 Minutes

Servings: 20 blondies

Ingredients

2 tablespoons of walnuts

1/2 ounce of chopped dark chocolate

1/4 teaspoon of salt

1/4 teaspoon of baking soda

2 tablespoons of coconut flour

1/4 cup of almond flour

2 tablespoons of coconut cream

1 teaspoon of vanilla extract

1/2 cup of erythritol

2 large eggs

4 tablespoons of unsalted butter

6 tablespoons of cacao butter

Directions

Preheat oven to around 320 degrees F then coat a baking dish using parchment paper.

Place butter and cacao butter in a bowl then put in the microwave.

Let the mixture melt for around 1 ½ minutes then stir making sure that the mixture has no lumps.

If required, you can microwave the mixture for an extra minute until it is smooth then put aside.

In a bowl, combine vanilla extract, erytritol and eggs with a hand mixer then put in coconut cream and combine again.

Add in the butter mixture and combine until mixture is creamy and dense then sieve coconut flour and almond flour.

Mix salt, baking soda and the flours then add this mixture to cream mixture and mix well using a spatula.

Put in chocolate and mix again then add in walnuts, orchia seeds or any other types of nuts that you like together with one teaspoon of lemon zest.

You can add the nuts to the chocolate or use alone then mix with a spatula.

Place mixture into the coated baking dish and evenly spread it out with a spatula then place in the preheated oven for about 30 minutes.

Use a toothpick or knife to test whether it is ready; it is when it comes out clean when inserted at the middle.

It is however not important that the toothpick is entirely clean as the blondies should be a bit fudgy at the centre.

Do not overcook the blondies.

Once you are done with cooking the blondies, remove from the pan together with parchment paper.

Leave it to cool then slice into equally sized blondies.

Nutritional Information Per Serving (One blondie): 80 Calories, 7.3 grams fats, 1.6 grams carbs, 2.1 grams proteins

Berry Bomb Pops

Prep Time: 20 Minutes

Cook Time: 3 Hours 30 Minutes

Total Time: 3 Hours 50 Minutes

Servings: 6 pops

Ingredients

Popsicle moulds and sticks

½ teaspoon of vanilla extract

1 ½ cups of canned coconut cream

1 ½ teaspoons of liquid stevia, divided

1 cup of water, divided

1 cup of frozen blueberries

1 cup of frozen raspberries

Directions

Put in a skillet 1/2 teaspoon of stevia, 1/2 cup of water and raspberries then let mixture boil on medium to high heat.

Boil for around 5 minutes or until fruits begin to remove some juice and some of liquid has reduced.

Remove the skillet from heat then transfer the mixture to a blender and blend until you get a smooth mixture.

Place the mixture in a bowl and put in a fridge.

Repeat this for blueberries.

Put 1/2 teaspoon of stevia, 1/2 cup of water and blue berries in a skillet on medium to high heat.

Boil the mixture for around 5 minutes.

Remove the skillet from heat and place the mixture in a blender.

Blend until you get a smooth puree then put aside in a fridge for it to cool until when you want to use it.

As the raspberry and blueberry mixtures are in the fridge, combine together vanilla extract, 1/2 teaspoon of stevia and coconut cream.

Stir until well combined then put aside in fridge.

To make popsicles, begin by equally dividing raspberry mixture into moulds.

Add carefully about two to three tablespoons of raspberry mixture at the middle of every mould, filling around one thirds full.

Put moulds in a freezer and let it chill for about one hour until it sets.

Equally divide the coconut mixture into moulds using same spoon around three to four tablespoons in every mould.

Make sure you work fast to avoid raspberry mixture bleeding to coconut mixture.

Put back into freezer until it partially sets for around 30 minutes.

This time make sure you time the popsicles.

The coconut mixture will be firm enough to hold popsicle skewers but still soft that the skewers can be inserted.

Put one stick into every mould leaving some stick at the top for holding the popsicles.

Put back in freezer for another hour until entirely solid.

Once solid, divide the blueberry mixture among the moulds with a spoon around two to three tablespoons in every mould.

Put back in the freezer for another one to two hours until it sets completely.

Enjoy.

Nutritional Information Per Serving: 146.33 Calories, 13.07 grams fats, 5.26 grams carbs, 1.14 grams proteins

Pecan Ice Cream

Prep Time: 2 Hours 10 Minutes

Cook Time: 40 Minutes

Total Time: 2 Hours 50 Minutes

Servings: 8

Ingredients

2 tablespoons of toasted and chopped pecans

1 tablespoons of MCT oil

1 tablespoons of maple pecan sweetener

2 teaspoons of maple extract

2 egg yolks

1/4 teaspoon of salt

1/2 cup of Swerve sweetener confectioners

2 cups of heavy cream

1/4 cup of butter

Directions

In a pan, on low heat, melt butter, salt, swerve sweetener and heavy cream then mix egg yolks in a bowl.

Mix well until the eggs have a light colour.

Scoop with a spoon the egg mixture and add into the butter mixture.

Continue adding spoonfuls of the egg mixture into butter mixture then add gradually the rest of the yolk mixture.

Let the mixture boil while stirring frequently until the mixture coats back of a spoon and becomes thick.

Transfer to a medium bowl and place in the fridge for around 30 minutes.

Put in MCT oil, swerve sweetener and maple extract and combine well then add the mixture to an ice cream maker.

Once ready, add in pecans and spread the ice cream in a loaf pan then place in the freezer for around 2-3 hours.

Nutritional Information Per Serving: 302 Calories, 32 grams fats, 2 grams carbs, 2 grams proteins

Chocolate With Berries And Cream

Prep Time: 15 Minutes

Cook Time: 20 Minutes

Total Time: 35 Minutes

Servings: 16

Ingredients

Dark chocolate cake

1 teaspoon of vanilla extract

1 pinch of salt

5 eggs

5 ounces of butter

9 ounces of dark chocolate with a minimum of 70% cocoa solids

For serving

2 cups of crème fraîche

½ cup of unsweetened coconut chips, roasted

4 ounces of chopped pecans

6 tablespoons of lime juice

1 teaspoon of vanilla extract

2 cups of fresh raspberries

Directions

Preheat oven to around 320 degrees then grease spring form about 9 inches in diameter with some coconut oil or butter.

Coat the form with some parchment paper at the bottom then break chocolate into small pieces and cut the butter into a cube.

Place these in a microwave safe bowl and put in microwave for a few minutes on low power while stirring frequently.

Make sure you are careful as chocolate burns if you do not stir constantly.

Leave the mixture to cool a few minutes.

Separate egg whites and egg yolks and place in different bowls then put some salt into egg whites and beat until you form a stiff peak. Put aside.

Put vanilla into the egg yolks and mix until the mixture is smooth.

Add butter and chocolate mixture into egg yolk and combine well then fold in egg whites.

Continue folding the mixture until you are no longer able to see white streaks from egg whites.

Add the batter into prepared spring form and bake for about 15-20 minutes then insert a knife or toothpick at the middle of the cake.

If it comes out clean then the cake is ready. Make sure the cake is not runny but moist.

Combine together vanilla, lime juice and berries in a mixing bowl and put aside for a couple of minutes.

Add cream into a bowl and beat until it forms a soft peak then equally divide the cake using your fingers into biteable pieces and place on plates.

Put in berries and drizzle with some nuts and coconut flakes on top of the cake.

Serve right away with the cream or crème fraiche.

Nutritional Information Per Serving: 355 Calories, 32 grams fats, 9 grams carbs, 5 grams proteins

Coconut Raspberry Slice

Prep Time: 1Hour 20 Minutes

Cook Time: 15 Minutes

Total Time: 1 Hour 35 Minutes

Servings: 20 slices

Ingredients

For the biscuit layer

1 large egg

1 tablespoon of butter, room temperature

½ teaspoon of baking soda

2 cups of almond meal

For the coconut layer

Pinch of sea salt

1 teaspoon of vanilla bean powder

1/3 cup of powdered erythritol

3 cups of desiccated coconut

¼ cup of coconut oil

1 cup of coconut milk, unsweetened

For the raspberry layer

2 tablespoons of water

3 tablespoons of chia seeds

1 teaspoon of powdered erythritol

1 cup of raspberries

For the chocolate layer

4 ounces of 85% dark chocolate

Directions

Preheat oven to about 350 degrees F then in a mixing bowl, mix well all of the biscuit ingredients until you form a dough.

Coat a brownie sheet or baking pan with some parchment paper then press evenly biscuit batter into the coated dish until you form a base.

Bake for about 15 minutes until browned lightly and cooked well before leaving it to cool.

Prepare raspberry by combining together all of the ingredients in a pan on low heat and stir to combine.

Break the raspberries up to make some jam then continue to stir for about 5 minutes until the mixture is thick; let it cool.

Combine coconut oil and coconut milk in a saucepan on medium heat and stir until well combined then mix the rest of the ingredients for making coconut layer.

Put in the oil and coconut milk mixture into dry ingredients and mix well.

Add in coconut mix to the biscuit base and evenly spread the mixture then put in a fridge until the mixture sets for about one hour.

After coconut layer hardens, pour raspberry mixture on top and put back into freezer for about one hour to set.

Break chocolate into tiny pieces, put in a bowl and place in the microwave.

Melt the chocolate for about 3 minutes and pour it over raspberry then place back in the fridge until the chocolate sets.

Remove it from fridge after about 30 minutes before you serve as it makes it quite easy to slice.

Cut into slices and place in fridge for about one week or in freezer for about 3 months.

Nutritional Information Per Serving: 241.53 Calories, 22.17 grams fats, 3.54 grams carbs, 4.64 grams proteins

Chia Seed Pudding

Prep Time: 10 Minutes

Cook Time: 1 Hour

Total Time: 1 Hour 10 Minutes

Servings: 4

Ingredients

1/4 cup of dark chocolate chips, sugar-free

2 tablespoons of crushed roasted almonds

1/3 cup of chia seeds

1 teaspoon of pure vanilla extract

1/4 cup of powered erytritol

1/4 cup of unsweetened cocoa powder

1/2 cup of unsweetened coconut flakes divided

2 cups of almond milk, unsweetened

Directions

In a blender, combine vanilla extract, erythritol, cocoa powder, a half of the coconut flakes and milk.

Blend until all the ingredients are well mixed then put mixture in a large bowl.

Put in chia seeds and mix well for about 1-2 minutes then serve the pudding in cups or bowls and place in a refrigerator for about 1-2 hours.

Garnish with chocolate chips, remaining coconut flakes, and almonds.

Nutritional Information Per Serving: 172 Calories, 12.3 grams fats, 12.8 grams carbs, 6.5 grams proteins

Matcha Skillet Souffle

Prep Time: 10 Minutes

Cook Time: 15 Minutes

Total Time: 25 Minutes

Servings: 1

Ingredients

¼ cup of whipped cream

1 tablespoon of unsweetened cocoa powder

1 tablespoon of coconut oil

7 whole raspberries

1 tablespoon of butter

1 tablespoon of matcha powder

1 teaspoon of vanilla extract

2 tablespoons of Swerve confectioners

3 large eggs

Directions

Preheat oven then place a skillet on medium heat and separate egg yolks from egg whites.

Beat egg whites and swerve confectioners then when a soft peak forms, put in matcha powder.

Whisk the mixture until a stiff peak forms then use a fork to beat the yolks in another bowl.

Put in vanilla and a little amount of egg whites then fold in carefully the remaining egg whites into yolk mix.

Place one tablespoon of the butter in a saucepan on medium heat and leave it to melt then add in soufflé mix.

Reduce heat and put raspberries over the soufflé then leave it to cook until the eggs are set.

Transfer the skillet to preheated oven and carefully watch it then remove from the oven after the top begins to brown.

Make sure not to leave the soufflé in the oven for so long as it might burn or turn dark.

In another pan on low heat, melt some coconut oil then add in cocoa powder and the rest of the swerve confectioners.

Serve the soufflé with a quarter cup of the whipped cream and sprinkle with confectioner's mixture.

Nutritional Information Per Serving: 578 Calories, 50.91 grams fats, 5.06 grams carbs, 20.95 grams proteins

Keto Flan

Prep Time: 4 Hours 20 Minutes

Cook Time: 35 Minutes

Total Time: 4 Hours 55 Minutes

Servings: 4

Ingredients

¼ cup of erythritol, for custard

1 tablespoon of vanilla

2 large egg yolks

2 large eggs

1 cup of heavy whipping cream

1 tablespoon of butter

⅛ cup of water

⅓ cup of erythritol, for caramel

Directions

In a saucepan, heat erytritol for caramel and mix it regularly.

Put in butter and water and mix occasionally until the sauce is golden brown.

Add the mixture at the bottom of every ramekin ensuring to cover the bottom well then put aside and let the mixture cool.

In a mixing bowl, combine together vanilla, left erytritol and whipping cream then in another bowl, beat together the eggs.

Add into the eggs the yolks and mix again.

Gently mix in the egg mixture into cream mixture then pour the mixture into every ramekin over caramel.

Put ramekins in a baking dish and halfway fill the dish with some hot water.

Bake for about 30 minutes at 350 degrees F.

Remove the baking dish from the oven; however, leave ramekins in hot water for an extra 10 minutes.

Remove the ramekins from the dish and leave them to sit in a fridge for about 4 hours or overnight.

Once ready, run a knife gently around the sides of custard to remove it from ramekin then turn upside down the ramekin.

Gently jiggle custard on a plate, serve and enjoy.

Nutritional Information Per Serving: 298 Calories, 31.5 grams fats, 2.4 grams carbs, 4.5 grams proteins

Bacon Asparagus Bites

Prep Time: 10 Minutes

Cook Time: 20 Minutes

Total Time: 30 Minutes

Servings: 6

Ingredients

9 blanched asparagus spears

Kosher salt

Freshly ground black pepper

1 minced garlic clove

5 ounces of softened cream cheese

6 slices of bacon, sliced into thirds

Directions

Preheat oven to about 400 degrees and coat a baking mat with some parchment paper.

Make the bacon by heating a pan on medium heat and cook the bacon until most the bacon fat has evaporated but not crispy.

Remove bacon from pan and drain them on a plate lined with paper towel.

In a mixing bowl, mix together garlic and cream cheese then season with some pepper and salt before mixing until well combined.

Spread around a half tablespoon of cream cheese on a piece of bacon then put spears at the centre and roll the bacon until the ends meet.

Repeat this for all of the spears and put on a baking mat then bake for about 5 minutes until cream cheese heats through and the bacon is crispy.

Nutritional Information Per Serving: 343 Calories, 27.4 grams fats, 2.91 grams carbs, 20.77 grams proteins

Parmesan Crisps

Prep Time: 10 Minutes

Cook Time: 9 Minutes

Total Time: 19 Minutes

Servings:

Ingredients

1 medium Jalapeno

2 slices of Provolone Cheese

8 tablespoons of parmesan cheese, grated

Directions

On a parchment paper or baking sheet, create eight 1 tablespoon scoops of parmesan about one inch from each other.

Cut jalapeno as thick or thin as you want then place them on the baking sheet or parchment paper and bake for around 5 minutes at 425 degrees F.

After jalapenos are ready and have cooled for a few minutes, put over each scoop of parmesan, pressing down slightly.

Split every provolone cheese into four pieces to make eight in total then place them over the parmesan and jalapeno.

Bake for 9 minutes at 425 F.

Nutritional Information Per Serving: 162 Calories, 10 grams fats, 1.5 grams carbs, 14 grams proteins

Keto Popcorn

Prep Time: 5 Minutes

Cook Time: 0 Minutes

Total Time: 5 Minutes

Servings: 2 cups

Ingredients

¾ teaspoons of five spice powder

1 teaspoon of grey sea salt

1¼ pounds (570 g) of pork belly, sliced into 1 by ½ inch pieces

½ cup of coconut oil

Sticky sauce, optional

½ teaspoon of fresh ginger, diced finely

½ teaspoon of garlic powder

1 teaspoon of erythritol

1 tablespoon of coconut aminos

2 teaspoons of sriracha

¼ cup of avocado oil

⅓ cup of pork stock

Directions

Put some oil in a skillet over medium to high heat then put in pork pieces in salt and after the oil completely melts, put in pork.

Cover and cook for around 20 minutes rotating the pieces when halfway through.

Once ready, strain the pork and you can reserve the bacon fat to use another time.

In the meantime, mix all of the remaining ingredients in a pan over medium to low heat.

Mix and let the mixture boil for about 10 minutes, mixing after 2 minutes.

Place the sauce in a small bowl and serve with the popcorn.

Nutritional Information Per Serving: 884 Calories, 64.6 grams fats, 0 grams carbs, 65.8 grams proteins

Smoked Salmon and Goat Cheese Bites

Prep Time: 20 Minutes

Cook Time: 0 Minutes

Total Time: 20 Minutes

Servings: 16 Cheese Bites

Ingredients

4 ounces of smoked salmon

3.9 ounces of radicchio

Salt and pepper to taste

2 cloves of garlic

1 tablespoon of fresh basil

1 tablespoon of fresh rosemary

1 tablespoon of fresh oregano

8 ounces of softened goat cheese

Directions

Mince finely basil, rosemary and oregano then grate finely garlic and put pepper, salt, garlic, herbs and goat cheese in a bowl.

Mix well and put aside.

Slice off the stems from bottom part of radicchio then peel carefully the leaves apart until there is only 16 leaves to be used for serving.

If you like, you can use any of the remaining radicchio to make other salad recipes.

Wash and dry the radicchio leaves then place a piece of salmon on each of the leaves together with ½ ounce of goat cheese.

Drizzle with some pepper and serve.

Nutritional Information Per Serving: 46.19 Calories, 3.33 grams fats, 0.94 grams carbs, 3.43 grams proteins

Zucchini Nacho Chips

Prep Time: 5 Minutes

Cook Time: 20 Minutes

Total Time: 25 Minutes

Servings: 4

Ingredients

1 tablespoon of Tex-Mex seasoning

1½ cups of coconut oil

Salt

1 large zucchini

Directions

Slice zucchini with a mandolin vertically into slices then put the zucchini slices in the colander in sink.

Drizzle with a lot of salt and leave them to sit for around 5 minutes before pressing out for any water.

Heat some oil in a pan to about 350 degrees F or 180 degrees C then add into the oil the zucchini in portions of around 20 chips each time.

After the zucchini becomes brown, remove from the pan and put on a paper towel.

Drizzle with some taco seasoning.

Nutritional Information Per Serving: 145 Calories, 14 grams fats, 2 grams carbs, 1 grams proteins

Chocolate Chip Granola Bars

Prep Time: 10 Minutes

Cook Time: 25 Minutes

Total Time: 35 Minutes

Servings: 16 bars

Ingredients

1/2 teaspoon of vanilla extract

1/2 cup of powdered Swerve Sweetener

1 tablespoon of Sukrin gold fibre syrup

1/2 cup of butter

1/2 teaspoon of salt

1/3 cup of sugar-free chocolate chips

1/3 cup of dried, unsweetened and chopped cranberries

1/2 cup of sunflower seeds

1/2 cup of pecan halves

1 cup of almonds, sliced

1 cup of flaked coconut

Direction

Preheat oven to around 300 degrees F and coat an 8*8 inch dish with some parchment paper leaving some excess parchment hanging on the edges of the dish.

In a processor, combine together sunflower seeds, pecans, almonds and coconut then blend on high speed until the mixture looks like coarse crumbs.

Transfer mixture to a bowl and mix in salt, chips and cranberries then in a skillet, on low heat, melt butter together with the fibre syrup.

After the butter melts, mix in sweetener until the mixture is smooth then put in vanilla extract.

Mix in the butter mix into the coconut mix until well mixed then pour the mixture into the coated baking dish and even it out.

Using a measuring cup, press the batter down until it is very compact then bake for about 25 minutes until the sides are browned.

Leave it to completely cool then with the excess parchment paper, lift it out.

Use a sharp knife to cut into bars and serve.

Nutritional Information Per Serving: 179 Calories, 16.32 grams fats, 6.24 grams carbs, 2.88 grams proteins

Tropical Smoothie

Prep Time: 5 Minutes

Cook Time: 0 Minutes

Total Time: 5 Minutes

Servings: 1

Ingredients

¼ teaspoon of banana extract

¼ teaspoon of blueberry extract

½ teaspoon of mango extract

20 drops of liquid Stevia

1 tablespoon of MCT Oil

2 tablespoons of golden flaxseed meal

¼ cup of sour cream

¾ cup of unsweetened coconut milk

7 large ice cubes

Directions

Put in all of the ingredients in a blender then wait for a couple of minutes to give the flax meal time to soak up some moisture.

Blend for around 1-2 minutes until all the ingredients are well incorporated then serve and enjoy.

Nutritional Information Per Serving: 355.75 Calories, 32.63 grams fats, 4.41 grams carbs, 4.4 grams proteins

Asparagus Fries

Prep Time: 10 Minutes

Cook Time: 10 Minutes

Total Time: 20 Minutes

Servings: 2

Ingredients

1 tablespoon of chopped finely roasted red pepper

3 tablespoons of mayonnaise

2 large eggs

½ teaspoon of smoked paprika

¼ cup of almond flour

½ teaspoon of garlic powder

2 tablespoons of chopped parsley

½ cup of shredded Parmesan cheese

10 medium asparagus spears

Directions

Preheat the oven to about 425 degrees F then wash asparagus spears.

In a processor, mix together garlic powder, parsley and parmesan cheese then blend until smooth.

Put in almond flour and blend around once or twice until the mixture combines well.

Place the mixture in a dish and mix in paprika.

In a bowl, whisk two eggs until frothy; make sure the eggs are frothy as they will stick better on asparagus.

Transfer the egg mixture to a shallow bowl.

Dip the asparagus in the egg mix then while holding the asparagus over the parmesan mix, drizzle gently the mixture as you turn it until coated lightly.

Ensure that the spears do not touch the parmesan mix, as the egg mixture will make the spear very clumpy and moist.

Repeat this with every asparagus.

Put the spear on a baking dish spaced tightly and garnish with the remaining parmesan mixture.

Bake for around 10 minutes until the spear is slightly soft and the coating on it starts to brown.

In a bowl, combine together mayonnaise and red pepper then place the mixture in a refrigerator to let the flavours to mix well.

Mix the mixture well before serving.

After the spear fries are brown and crisp, remove from oven and serve right away with the red pepper mixture.

Nutritional Information Per Serving: 453.65 Calories, 33.43 grams fats, 5.51 grams carbs, 19.14 grams proteins

Savory Spiced Pecans

Prep Time: 5 Minutes

Cook Time: 15 Minutes

Total Time: 20 Minutes

Servings: 8

Ingredients

1/4 teaspoon of cayenne pepper, if you want it spicy

1/4 cup of extra virgin olive oil

1/4 teaspoon of onion powder

2 teaspoons of fresh lemon zest

2 teaspoon of pink Himalayan salt

1/4 teaspoon of smoked paprika

1/4 teaspoon of garlic powder

4 tablespoons of fresh rosemary, chopped roughly

4 cups of pecans

Directions

Preheat the oven to around 180 degrees C then put the nuts in a mixing bowl and add in all of the spices apart from lemon zest.

Put in some olive oil and combine thoroughly the mixture until the nuts are equally coated.

Pour the mixture on a coated baking tray and spread evenly over the tray then bake for about 10-15 minutes until toasty and golden brown.

Mix the nuts after every five minutes to ensure equal browning; however, make sure you look after the nuts the last half of their cooking time to avoid burning.

Remove from the oven and leave them to slightly cool then drizzle with lemon zest on top.

Combine well and let the nuts completely cool then keep in air tight containers.

Nutritional Information Per Serving (½ cup): 348 Calories, 36.1 grams fats, 7.3 grams carbs, 4.6 grams proteins

Chia Seed Crackers

Prep Time: 20 Minutes

Cook Time: 35 Minutes

Total Time: 55 Minutes

Servings: yields 36 crackers

Ingredients

¼ teaspoon of pepper

¼ teaspoon of salt

¼ teaspoon of paprika

¼ teaspoon of oregano

¼ teaspoon of onion powder

¼ teaspoon of garlic powder

¼ teaspoon of xanthan gum

2 tablespoons of olive oil

2 tablespoons of psyllium husk powder

1 ¼ cups of ice water

3 ounces of cheddar cheese, shredded

½ cup of ground chia seeds

Directions

Grind the chia seeds in a grinder then mix together all of the dry ingredients in a mixing bowl.

Preheat oven to about 375 degrees and put in some olive oil into dry ingredients giving the mixture a wet and sandy consistency.

Add in some water into the mixture and combine well until you make a solid dough.

Put in cheddar cheese and with your hands, combine the mixture well then place on a baking mat to sit for a couple of minutes.

Roll out the dough into the size of a baking mat ensuring at it is very tin.

Bake for about 30-35 minutes then remove from oven and slice into crackers.

Return the crackers back in the oven for another 5-7 minutes until the crackers are crisp at the top and then leave them to cool then serve.

Nutritional Information Per Serving: 28.17 Calories, 2.15 grams fats, 0.28 grams carbs, 0.88 grams proteins

Bacon and Brussels Sprout Skewers

Prep Time: 10 Minutes

Cook Time: 25 Minutes

Total Time: 35 Minutes

Servings: Makes about 18 skewers

Ingredients

Small wooden skewers

1/4 teaspoon of sea salt

1 teaspoon of garlic powder

1 teaspoon of ghee

2 pounds of Brussels sprouts

1 pound of bacon

Directions

Slice the strips of bacon into two horizontally then in a skillet, over medium heat, fry bacon until it is almost cooked but still a bit soft.

Ensure that you do not overcook the bacon, as this will make is hard to put onto the wooden skewer.

Remove bacon from skillet and put aside on a plate then get rid of almost all the bacon fat retaining enough to coat the pan.

Slice the Brussels horizontally into two and put sea salt, garlic powder, ghee and sprouts into the pan.

Fry for a few minutes over medium heat until the sprouts are soft and brown then preheat an oven to around 375 degrees F.

Put one end of bacon onto the end of the wooden skewer then add in a sprout slice and weave bacon round sprout and back again through the wooden skewer, making sure that you make a wave pattern between sprouts.

Move sprout and bacon down the wooden skewer and repeat this about 2-3 times for every skewer.

Bake for about 5-10 minutes in a baking sheet until the bacon is cooked well.

Nutritional Information Per Serving: 151 Calories, 11 grams fats, 2.8 grams carbs, 10.2 grams proteins

Cheesy Bacon Stuffed Mini Peppers

Prep Time: 15 Minutes

Cook Time: 12 Minutes

Total Time: 27 Minutes

Servings: 12

Ingredients

Chopped cilantro for topping

1 teaspoon of Worcestershire sauce

1/2 cup of cheddar cheese, shredded plus extra for topping

1/2 teaspoon of garlic powder

4 slices of cooked and crumbled bacon

2 Tablespoons of sliced green onions

4 ounces of cream cheese

6 mini sweet peppers cut in half, seeds and membranes removed

Directions

Preheat oven to about 400 degrees then coat a baking sheet with some cooking spray and put aside.

In a bowl, mix together, using an electric mixer, Worcestershire sauce, cheddar, garlic powder, bacon, green onions and cream cheese.

Combine until smooth.

Scoop a tablespoon of the filling and put in the peppers then place on the cookie sheet.

Drizzle each of the peppers with some more cheese then bake in the oven for about 10-12 minutes until the cheese is bubbly and has melted and the peppers become soft.

Leave them to cool and garnish with cilantro.

Nutritional Information Per Serving: 87 Calories, 7 grams fats, 1 grams carbs, 2 grams proteins

Keto Meal Plan for 90 Days

Week 1

Monday

- **Breakfast:** Keto rolls

- **Lunch:** Eggplant and Beef Casserole

- **Dinner:** Chicken Cacciatore

- **Snack/dessert:** Vegan Coconut Macaroons

Tuesday

- **Breakfast:** Keto frittata

- **Lunch:** Leftovers of the Chicken Cacciatore

- **Dinner:** Cajun Shrimp Skillet

- **Dessert:** Keto Mocha Mousse

Wednesday

- **Breakfast:** Coconut cream with berries

- **Lunch:** Keto Lasagna Stuffed Portobellos

- **Dinner:** Keto Tortang Talong

- **Dessert:** Orange Cake Balls

Thursday

- **Breakfast:** Chorizo Omelette

- **Lunch:** Grilled Turkey Burger
- **Dinner:** Eggplant and Pork
- **Dessert:** Vegan coconut macaroons

Friday

- **Breakfast:** Bacon Cheeseburger Waffles
- **Lunch:** Keto Taco Bowls with Cauliflower Rice
- **Dinner:** Stuffed Meatloaf
- **Dessert:** Cacao butter keto blondies

Saturday

- **Breakfast:** Blueberry smoothie
- **Lunch:** Leftovers from the Keto stuffed Meatloaf
- **Dinner:** Chicken and Sausage Jambalaya
- **Dessert:** Berry Bomb Pops

Sunday

- **Breakfast:** Cream Cheese Pancake
- **Lunch:** Pork Skewers with Chimichurri
- **Dinner:** Bacon Wrapped Chicken Bombs
- **Dessert:** Pecan Ice Cream

Week 2

Monday

- **Breakfast:** Breakfast Biscuit Sandwiches

- **Lunch:** Keto Tortang Talong

- **Dinner:** Cajun Shrimp Skillet

- **Dessert:** Chocolate with berries and cream

Tuesday

- **Breakfast:** Keto Breakfast Cheesecake

- **Lunch:** Leftovers from the previous night

- **Dinner:** Rogan Josh

- **Dessert:** Coconut Raspberry Slice

Wednesday

- **Breakfast:** Low-carb cauliflower hash browns

- **Lunch:** Cheesy Zucchini Aglio e Olio

- **Dinner:** Stuffed Meatloaf

- **Dessert:** Chia Seed Pudding

Thursday

- **Breakfast:** Baked Mini-Frittatas

- **Lunch:** Mustard Chicken Recipe with Radishes and Spinach

- **Dinner:** Seafood Soup

- **Dessert:** Matcha Skillet Souffle

Friday

- **Breakfast:** Blueberry Smoothie

- **Lunch:** Chicken Stir Fry

- **Dinner:** Keto Shrimp Scampi

- **Dessert:** Pecan ice cream

Saturday

- **Breakfast:** Egg-Crust Breakfast Pizza

- **Lunch:** Dill pickle soup

- **Dinner:** Keto Shrimp Scampi

- **Dessert:** Keto Flan

Sunday

- **Breakfast:** Breakfast Roll Ups

- **Lunch:** Keto Dill Pickle Soup

- **Dinner:** Low-Carb Cauli Cottage Pie

- **Dessert:** Keto mocha mousse

Week 3

Monday

- **Breakfast:** Brie & Apple Crepes
- **Lunch:** Leftovers from the Low-Carb Cauli Cottage Pie
- **Dinner:** Lime Pork Chops
- **Dessert:** Chocolate with berries and cream

Tuesday

- **Breakfast:** Breakfast Salad
- **Lunch:** Caramelized Onion Croquettes Stuffed w/ Goat Cheese
- **Dinner:** Slow-Cooker Beef & Broccoli
- **Dessert:** Matcha Skillet Souffle

Wednesday

- **Breakfast:** Avocado Egg Bowls
- **Lunch:** Coleslaw-Stuffed Keto Wraps
- **Dinner:** Cashew Chicken
- **Dessert:** Pecan ice cream

Thursday

- **Breakfast:** Sausage Gravy and Biscuit Bake

- **Lunch:** Leftovers from the Cashew chicken

- **Dinner:** Chicken stir fry

- **Dessert:** Keto flan

Friday

- **Breakfast:** Chicken and Zucchini Breakfast Quiche

- **Lunch:** Leftovers from the Chicken stir-fry

- **Dinner:** Keto Salmon Curry

- **Dessert:** Cranberry Chocolate Chip Granola Bars

Saturday

- **Breakfast:** Pumpkin Spice Latte

- **Lunch:** Keto Reuben skillet

- **Dinner:** Broccoli Beef

- **Dessert:** Tropical Smoothie

Sunday

- **Breakfast:** Coconut cream with berries

- **Lunch:** Leftovers from the Broccoli Beef

- **Dinner:** Lemon and Dill Pan Seared Salmon

- **Dessert:** Matcha Skillet Souffle

Week 4

Monday

- **Breakfast:** Crustless Quiche
- **Lunch:** Beef Satay and Peanut Sauce
- **Dinner:** Salmon Curry
- **Dessert:** Chia Seed Pudding

Tuesday

- **Breakfast:** Cream Cheese Pancake
- **Lunch:** Mini Meatloaves
- **Dinner:** Salmon with Tomato Cream Sauce
- **Dessert:** Coconut Raspberry Slice

Wednesday

- **Breakfast:** Basic Oopsie Rolls
- **Lunch:** Sesame Salmon w. Baby Bok Choy & Mushrooms
- **Dinner:** Keto Beef Bulgogi
- **Dessert:** Pecan ice cream

Thursday

- **Breakfast:** Breakfast Salad
- **Lunch:** Greek Meatballs Salad

- **Dinner:** Lemon and Dill Pan Seared Salmon

- **Dessert:** Chocolate, berries with cream

Friday

- **Breakfast:** Egg-Crust Breakfast Pizza with Pepperoni, Olives, Mozzarella, and Tomatoes

- **Lunch:** Leftovers from the Creamy Lemon and Dill Pan Seared Salmon

- **Dinner:** Bacon Wrapped Chicken Bombs

- **Dessert:** Matcha skillet souffle

Saturday

- **Breakfast:** Keto Cinnamon Rolls

- **Lunch:** Keto Broccoli Soup with Turmeric and Ginger

- **Dinner:** Crispy Skin Salmon with Pesto Cauliflower Rice

- **Dessert:** Keto Mocha Mousse

Sunday

- **Breakfast:** BBQ Bacon Cheeseburger Waffles

- **Lunch:** Low-Carb Zucchini Nachos

- **Dinner:** Easy Chicken Cacciatore

- **Dessert:** Coconut raspberry slice

Week 5

Monday

- **Breakfast:** Keto Breakfast Cheesecake
- **Lunch:** Chicken Nuggets
- **Dinner:** Spicy Eggplant and Minced Pork
- **Dessert:** Tropical smoothie

Tuesday

- **Breakfast:** Cauliflower hash browns
- **Lunch:** Low Carb Chicken Philly Cheesesteak
- **Dinner:** Cajun Shrimp Skillet
- **Dessert:** Orange Cake Balls

This 30 day meal plan is enough to get you in ketosis and enable you to lose several pounds with great ease. But what if you want to continue? Is there a way you can follow the recipes we've discussed for more than the 30 days; perhaps 60 days or 90 days? I thought you may want an extended version of the meal plan, which is why I have a bonus to take you for another 2 months. Let's get to that.

Keto Meal Plan

Bonus Meal Plan If You Are Hooked To The Keto Diet

Week 5 Continued

Wednesday

- **Breakfast:** Breakfast Biscuit Sandwiches

- **Lunch:** Leftovers from the Low Carb Chicken Philly Cheesesteak

- **Dinner:** Bacon Wrapped Chicken Bombs

- **Dessert:** Cacao butter keto blondies

Thursday

- **Breakfast:** Baked Mini-Frittatas

- **Lunch:** Keto Tortang Talong

- **Dinner:** Chicken and Sausage Jambalaya

- **Dessert:** Pecan Ice Cream

Friday

- **Breakfast:** Blueberry smoothie

- **Lunch:** Easy Asiago Cauliflower Rice

- **Dinner:** Bacon Wrapped Chicken Bombs

- **Dessert:** Berry Bomb Pops

Saturday

- **Breakfast:** Chorizo Omelette

- **Lunch:** Healthy Turkey Lettuce Wraps

- **Dinner:** Rogan Josh

- **Dessert:** Coconut Raspberry Slice

Sunday

- **Breakfast:** Keto frittata

- **Lunch:** Stuffed Bell Peppers

- **Dinner:** Keto Lime Pork Chops

- **Dessert:** Chocolate with berries and cream

Week 6

Monday

- **Breakfast:** Keto Rolls

- **Lunch:** Grilled Turkey Burger

- **Dinner:** Low-Carb Cauli Cottage Pie

- **Dessert:** Matcha Skillet Souffle

Tuesday

- **Breakfast:** Breakfast Salad

- **Lunch:** Chicken Stir Fry

- **Dinner:** Keto Stuffed Meatloaf

- **Dessert:** Chia Seed Pudding

Wednesday

- **Breakfast:** Breakfast Roll Ups

- **Lunch:** Leftovers from the chicken stir fry

- **Dinner:** Seafood Soup

- **Dessert:** Keto Flan

Thursday

- **Breakfast:** Chicken and Zucchini Breakfast Quiche

- **Lunch:** Eggplant and Beef Casserole

- **Dinner:** Keto Shrimp Scampi

- **Dessert:** Pistachio toffee cups

Friday

- **Breakfast:** Avocado Egg Bowls

- **Lunch:** Leftovers from the eggplant and beef casserole

- **Dinner:** Chicken and Sausage Jambalaya

- **Dessert:** Chocolate with berries and cream

Saturday

- **Breakfast:** Keto Sausage Gravy and Biscuit Bake

- **Lunch:** Easy Keto Lasagna Stuffed Portobellos

- **Dinner:** Keto Lime Pork Chops

- **Dessert:** Pistachio toffee cups

Sunday

- **Breakfast:** Pumpkin Spice Latte

- **Lunch:** Leftovers from the pork chops

- **Dinner:** Low-Carb Cauli Cottage Pie

- **Dessert:** Coconut raspberry slice

Week 7

Monday

- **Breakfast:** Coconut cream with berries
- **Lunch:** Keto Taco Bowls with Cauliflower Rice
- **Dinner:** Slow-Cooker Beef & Broccoli
- **Dessert:** Keto flan

Tuesday

- **Breakfast:** Instant Pot Crustless Quiche Lorraine
- **Lunch:** Leftovers from the beef and broccoli
- **Dinner:** Easy Cashew Chicken
- **Dessert:** Chia seed pudding

Wednesday

- **Breakfast:** Cream Cheese Pancake
- **Lunch:** Pork Skewers with Chimichurri
- **Dinner:** Keto stuffed meatloaf
- **Dessert:** Keto Tropical Smoothie

Thursday

- **Breakfast:** Basic Oopsie Rolls
- **Lunch:** Leftovers from the keto stuffed meatloaf

- **Dinner:** Keto Salmon Curry

- **Dessert:** Cranberry Chocolate Chip Granola Bars

Friday

- **Breakfast:** Keto Sausage Gravy and Biscuit Bake

- **Lunch:** Keto Tortang Talong

- **Dinner:** Chicken Cacciatore

- **Dessert:** Berry Bomb Pops

Saturday

- **Breakfast:** Egg-Crust Breakfast Pizza with Pepperoni, Olives, Mozzarella, and Tomatoes

- **Lunch:** Leftovers from the Easy Chicken Cacciatore

- **Dinner:** Easy Paleo Broccoli Beef

- **Dessert:** Coconut raspberry slice

Sunday

- **Breakfast:** Blueberry Coconut Porridge

- **Lunch:** Cheesy Zucchini Aglio e Olio

- **Dinner:** Eggplant and Minced Pork

- **Dessert:** Keto flan

Week 8

Monday

- **Breakfast:** Bacon Cheeseburger Waffles
- **Lunch:** Leftovers from the cheesy zucchini
- **Dinner:** Salmon with Pesto Cauliflower Rice
- **Dessert:** Chia seed pudding

Tuesday

- **Breakfast:** Cauliflower hash browns
- **Lunch:** Leftovers from the salmon and cauliflower rice
- **Dinner:** Keto Beef Bulgogi
- **Dessert:** Keto mocha mousse

Wednesday

- **Breakfast:** Almond Crusted Breakfast Keto Cheesecake
- **Lunch:** Grilled Turkey Burger
- **Dinner:** Creamy Lemon and Dill Pan Seared Salmon
- **Dessert:** Chocolate with berries and cream

Keto Meal Plan

Thursday

- **Breakfast:** Blueberry smoothie

- **Lunch:** Keto Mustard Chicken with Radishes and Spinach

- **Dinner:** Salmon with Bacon and Tomato Cream Sauce

- **Dessert:** Vegan Coconut Macaroons

Friday

- **Breakfast:** Breakfast Biscuit Sandwiches

- **Lunch:** Leftovers from the bacon and tomato cream sauce

- **Dinner:** Spicy Eggplant and Minced Pork

- **Dessert:** Keto Mocha Mousse

Saturday

- **Breakfast:** Baked Mini-Frittatas

- **Lunch:** Leftovers from the eggplant and pork

- **Dinner:** Cajun Shrimp Skillet

- **Dessert:** Orange Cake Balls

Sunday

- **Breakfast:** Chorizo Omelette

- **Lunch:** Dill Pickle Soup

- **Dinner:** Chicken Cacciatore

- **Dessert:** Pecan ice cream

Week 9

Monday

- **Breakfast:** Keto frittata
- **Lunch:** Leftovers from the pickle soup
- **Dinner:** Chicken and Sausage Jambalaya
- **Dessert:** Cacao butter keto blondies

Tuesday

- **Breakfast:** Avocado Egg Bowls
- **Lunch:** Chicken Nuggets
- **Dinner:** Rogan Josh
- **Dessert:** Berry Bomb Pops

Wednesday

- **Breakfast:** Pumpkin Spice Latte
- **Lunch:** Leftovers from Rogan Josh
- **Dinner:** Keto Shrimp Scampi
- **Dessert:** Pecan Ice Cream

Thursday

- **Breakfast:** Breakfast Salad

- **Lunch:** Caramelized Onion Croquettes Stuffed w/ Goat Cheese

- **Dinner:** Bacon Wrapped Chicken Bombs

- **Dessert:** Chocolate with berries and cream

Friday

- **Breakfast:** Chicken and Zucchini Breakfast Quiche

- **Lunch:** Coleslaw-Stuffed Keto Wraps

- **Dinner:** Keto Stuffed Meatloaf

- **Dessert:** Coconut Raspberry Slice

Saturday

- **Breakfast:** Brie & Apple Crepes

- **Lunch:** Leftovers from the meatloaf

- **Dinner:** Seafood Soup

- **Dessert:** Chia Seed Pudding

Sunday

- **Breakfast:** Coconut cream with berries

- **Lunch:** Beef Satay and Peanut Sauce

- **Dinner:** Keto Shrimp Scampi

- **Dessert:** Matcha Skillet Souffle

Week 10

Monday

- **Breakfast:** Sausage Gravy and Biscuit Bake

- **Lunch:** Keto Reuben skillet

- **Dinner:** Chicken and Sausage Jambalaya

- **Dessert:** Chocolate Chip Granola Bars

Tuesday

- **Breakfast:** Cream Cheese Pancake

- **Lunch:** Leftovers from the Keto Reuben skillet

- **Dinner:** Keto Lime Pork Chops

- **Dessert:** Keto Flan

Wednesday

- **Breakfast:** Cauliflower hash browns

- **Lunch:** Leftovers from the pork chops

- **Dinner:** Low-Carb Cauli Cottage Pie

- **Dessert:** Chocolate with berries and cream

Thursday

- **Breakfast:** Breakfast Biscuit Sandwiches

- **Lunch:** Leftovers from the cottage pie

- **Dinner:** Slow-Cooker Beef & Broccoli

- **Dessert:** Pecan ice cream

Friday

- **Breakfast:** Basic Oopsie Rolls

- **Lunch:** Veggie-Loaded Mini Meatloaves

- **Dinner:** Salmon with Bacon and Tomato Cream Sauce

- **Dessert:** Cranberry Chocolate Chip Granola Bars

Saturday

- **Breakfast:** Egg-Crust Breakfast Pizza

- **Lunch:** Sesame Salmon w. Baby Bok Choy & Mushrooms

- **Dinner:** Keto Beef Bulgogi

- **Dessert:** Berry Bomb Pops

Sunday

- **Breakfast:** Blueberry Coconut Porridge

- **Lunch:** Greek Meatballs Salad

- **Dinner:** Salmon with Pesto Cauliflower Rice

- **Dessert:** Matcha Skillet Souffle

Week 11

Monday

- **Breakfast:** Breakfast Biscuit Sandwiches

- **Lunch:** Leftovers from the Greek Meatballs salad

- **Dinner:** Leftovers from the salmon and pesto cauliflower rice

- **Dessert:** Cranberry Chocolate Chip Granola Bars

Tuesday

- **Breakfast:** Blueberry smoothie

- **Lunch:** Keto Broccoli Soup with Turmeric

- **Dinner:** Cashew Chicken

- **Dessert:** Keto Tropical Smoothie

Wednesday

- **Breakfast:** Keto frittata

- **Lunch:** Greek Meatballs Salad

- **Dinner:** Lemon and Dill Pan Seared Salmon

- **Dessert:** Chocolate Chip Granola Bars

Thursday

- **Breakfast:** Keto Rolls

- **Lunch:** Chicken Nuggets

- **Dinner:** Slow cooker beef & broccoli

- **Dessert:** Berry Bomb Pops

Friday

- **Breakfast:** Bacon Cheeseburger Waffles

- **Lunch:** Low Carb Chicken Philly Cheesesteak

- **Dinner:** Keto Salmon Curry

- **Dessert:** Chia Seed Pudding

Saturday

- **Breakfast:** Chorizo Omelette

- **Lunch:** Leftovers from the cheesesteak

- **Dinner:** Keto Beef Bulgogi

- **Dessert:** Pecan ice cream

Sunday

- **Breakfast:** Baked Mini-Frittatas

- **Lunch:** Stuffed Bell Peppers

- **Dinner:** Keto Beef Bulgogi

- **Dessert:** Keto flan

Week 12

Monday

- **Breakfast:** Keto Rolls
- **Lunch:** Eggplant and Beef Casserole
- **Dinner:** Salmon with Pesto Cauliflower Rice
- **Dessert:** Keto Mocha Mousse

Tuesday

- **Breakfast:** Breakfast Biscuit Sandwiches
- **Lunch:** Leftovers from the eggplant and beef casserole
- **Dinner:** Rogan Josh
- **Dessert:** Berry bomb pops

Wednesday

- **Breakfast:** Basic Oopsie Rolls
- **Lunch:** Pork Skewers with Chimichurri
- **Dinner:** Chicken Cacciatore
- **Dessert:** Berry Bomb Pops

Thursday

- **Breakfast:** Chorizo Omelette
- **Lunch:** Keto Tortang Talong

- **Dinner:** Low-Carb Cauli Cottage Pie

- **Dessert:** Pecan Ice Cream

Friday

- **Breakfast:** Breakfast Keto Cheesecake

- **Lunch:** Cheesy Zucchini Aglio e Olio

- **Dinner:** Keto Salmon Curry

- **Dessert:** Chocolate with berries and cream

Saturday

- **Breakfast:** Pumpkin Spice Latte

- **Lunch:** Lasagna Stuffed Portobello

- **Dinner:** Eggplant and Minced Pork

- **Dessert:** Coconut Raspberry Slice

Sunday

- **Breakfast:** Chicken and Zucchini Breakfast Quiche

- **Lunch:** Turkey Lettuce Wraps

- **Dinner:** Seafood Soup

- **Dessert:** Chia Seed Pudding

Week 13

Monday

- **Breakfast:** Breakfast Roll Ups
- **Lunch:** Low-Carb Zucchini Nachos
- **Dinner:** Lime Pork Chops
- **Dessert:** Matcha Skillet Souffle

Tuesday

- **Breakfast:** Breakfast Salad
- **Lunch:** Coleslaw-Stuffed Keto Wraps
- **Dinner:** Salmon with Tomato Cream Sauce
- **Dessert:** Easy Orange Cake Balls

Wednesday

- **Breakfast:** Crustless Quiche
- **Lunch:** Keto Reuben skillet
- **Dinner:** Keto Shrimp Scampi Recipe
- **Dessert:** Pecan ice cream

Thursday

- **Breakfast:** Blueberry Coconut Porridge
- **Lunch:** Dill Pickle Soup

- **Dinner:** Slow cooker beef and broccoli

- **Dessert:** Keto Flan

Friday

- **Breakfast:** Cauliflower hash browns

- **Lunch:** Mini Meatloaves

- **Dinner:** Salmon Curry

- **Dessert:** Keto Tropical Smoothie

Saturday

- **Breakfast:** Blueberry smoothie

- **Lunch:** Beef Satay and Peanut Sauce

- **Dinner:** Lemon and Dill Pan Seared Salmon

- **Dessert:** Cranberry Chocolate Chip Granola Bars

Sunday

- **Breakfast:** Keto frittata

- **Lunch:** Greek Meatballs Salad

- **Dinner:** Keto Beef Bulgogi

- **Dessert:** Berry bomb pops

You can eat any of the snacks in the book and you do not have to take dessert every day if you don't want to. Other snack options include nuts, seeds, deviled eggs, raw vegetables with dip cheese slices etc.

Conclusion

Thank you for taking the time to read this book.

I hope you now know quite a number of recipes that you can prepare in your kitchen and enjoy the keto lifestyle.

All the best in your quest for a healthier YOU.

Finally, I would like to ask you for a favour. Can you please leave a review for this book?

I will greatly appreciate that.

Thank you and Good Luck!

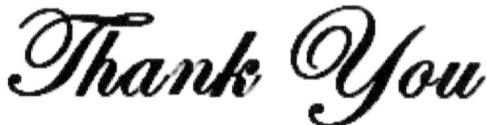

Printed in Great Britain
by Amazon